WHAT OTHERS ARE SAYING ...

"Weinstein approaches nutrition and exercise with military precision."

- The Miami Herald

"Bob spells out simple ways that need no gym or fancy gym equipment to get and stay in good physical shape .... Great job in writing this straight-forward message about the whole idea of life, being healthy and happy!"

- Ursula E. Hanks

"Highly motivating and interesting method for self-help in health & fitness. It concentrates on the affordable method, instead of spending lots of money on expensive equipment and gym fees to get fit. Includes how-to instruction, personal stories, and general guidance."

- Priscilla Smith

Col. Weinstein has been featured as a health and fitness expert:

Baptist Health Hospitals

Fitness Magazine

The History Channel

Fox Sports Net

The Washington Times

The Las Vegas Tribune

Eurosport, the largest European satellite and cable network

Gold Coast Magazine

Tropical Life Magazine

The Sun-sentinel

The Miami Herald

Many others

Most people never run far enough on their first wind to find out they've got a second. Give your dreams all you've got and you'll be amazed at the energy that comes out of you.

- William James, Psychologist and Author

BOOT CAMP
FITNESS
FOR ALL SHAPES AND SIZES

Complete Manual to Exceed Your Goals

The Health Colonel™ Series.

LCOL. Bob Weinstein, Ret.

TheHealthColonel.com

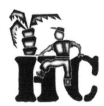

Boot Camp Fitness For All Shapes and Sizes: Complete Manual to Exceed Your Goals

By LCol. Bob Weinstein, Ret. (Lt. Col. Joseph R. Weinstein, USAR-Ret.)

TheHealthColonel.com

Categories: health and fitness, self-help, motivation

Copyright © 2010 by Lt. Col. Joseph R. Weinstein, USAR-Ret.

All Rights Reserved.

Publisher: The Health Colonel Publishing

ISBN-13: 978-0-9841783-1-5 Softcover

Unless otherwise indicated, all Scripture quotations are taken from the *Holy Bible,* New Living Translation, copyright © 1996. Used by permission of Tyndale House Publishers, Inc., Wheaton, Illinois 60189. All rights reserved.

First Edition 2008. Second Edition 2010, Revised

Before beginning any exercise program, consult your physician. The author and publisher of this book and workout disclaim any liability, personal or professional, resulting from the misapplication of any of the training instructions described in this publication.

Weinstein, Bob.
Weinstein, Joseph
Boot Camp Fitness For All Shapes and Sizes : complete guide to exceed your goals / by Bob Weinstein (Joseph Weinstein).– 2nd ed., rev.
Rev. ed. of: Change Made Easy. c2008
Includes bibliographical references and index.
ISBN-13: 978-0-9841783-1-5 (trade pbk. : alk. Paper)
1. Fitness–United States. I. Weinstein, Bob. Weinstein, Joseph. Boot Camp fitness. II. Title. III. Title: Boot Camp fitness

Printed in the United States

BOOT CAMP
FITNESS
FOR ALL SHAPES AND SIZES

Complete Manual to Exceed Your Goals

The Health Colonel™ Series.

LCol. Bob Weinstein, Ret.

TheHealthColonel.com

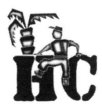

The successful person makes a habit of doing what the failing person doesn't like to do.

- Thomas Edison

Acknowledgments

Thank You…

To all my Beach Boot Camp recruits who have inspired me to write this book.

To the US Naval Sea Cadets, Team Spruance, Fort Lauderdale, FL and The Covenant House, Fort Lauderdale, Florida, the youth of both organizations have inspired me through their determination to improve their lives.

To David Miller, Superintendent of Parks and Recreation and the City of Fort Lauderdale for allowing me to use Fort Lauderdale Beach for Beach Boot Camp.

To Priscilla Smith for her diligent editing work.

To Denise Zacharias and Grit Gagelmann for their work demonstrating exercises.

To Andy Carrie for his great photography.

To Greg Gregory, Mikki Schneider, Priscilla Smith, Trudie Taylor Lou Taylor and Sarah Olsen for sharing their stories about weight loss and weight management.

To Brook Trace for her great photography.

To Gary Schwartz for his great photography.

In memory of
Mildred Weinstein,
my beloved grandmother "Gammie"
who passed away on
September 11, 2008

CONTENTS

PART ONE:

CHANGE YOUR LIFESTYLE - Ground Rules for Success

Introduction

"There are enemy soldiers on American soil. The names of these soldiers are Heart Disease, Cancer and Stroke. They are killing over 3,000 Americans a day." Lt. Col. Bob Weinstein, USAR-Ret.

You have in your hands a basic training book that will give you all the tools you need to take back control of your life and health. Basic training is foundational. The basics remain essential. Most decisions gone wrong have violated one or more basic principles. The basics of fitness and healthy living are no different. Follow these basics and you will have a strong foundation for health and fitness. **This new release includes a comprehensive index to make this basic training healthy lifestyle manual useful as a reference book and guide.** I will train you on the following topics:

How to exercise with little or no equipment.
How to manage your weight.

How to eat.

How to build strong character.

How to enhance performance and productivity.

How to get started on a spiritual journey and find your purpose.

How to save money and lives with a corporate wellness program.

How to establish goals and measure performance.

How to organize and implement your own fitness boot camp program.

Many of the tips and guidelines on eating and exercise are addressing our culture and society. If we were already predominantly leading an active lifestyle and eating a variety fruits, vegetables, nuts and grains in our diet, many of the health issues discussed would not be as prevalent.

Three basic diseases in this country and their death statistics were the catalyst behind *enemy soldiers*. The war in Iraq heightened my awareness about deaths caused by the enemy. The media has been focusing on constantly counting the number of soldiers killed while in the United States thousands of people die daily due to health-related preventable diseases.

Three diseases in particular -- namely heart disease, cancer and stroke -- kill over 3,000 Americans a day. Of those deaths, it is estimated that between 80 and 90 % are lifestyle related. This means there are reasonable, measurable and attainable healthy lifestyle changes that can be made which will result in a significant qualitatively improved life and greater longevity.

Of course there are many other diseases that are killing people due to how they live.

The truth is there are many "enemy soldiers" resulting in casualties and deaths in the United States and in other countries. These enemy soldiers are not just medical diseases. They begin with the very fabric of your interrelationships with your fellow man and woman. They begin with how you feel about yourself and others. They begin with the value you place on the lives and quality of lives of others. They begin with your taking personal responsibility for all that you say, do and think every day of your life whether driving in traffic or sitting at home alone. They begin with the understanding that everything you do, say and think has consequences for you and for others. You are not only personally responsible for all that you say, do and think; you are also a role model once you enter society and interact with others (or not).

Many times I will state -- yes shout -- a key question to those who attend my beach boot camp workouts on Fort Lauderdale Beach in South Florida,

"You may be saving two lives today. The first is your own. The second is the person who may observe you working out. Your presence working out may end up being the catalyst for someone leading a sedentary lifestyle to finally begin the journey of making healthy lifestyle changes and becoming active."

I had a conversation the other day about conspiracies. The individual I was speaking with was talking about all the alleged government conspiracies going on that negatively impact our lives.

Do we really need conspiratorial help from the government to sabotage our lives? Are we not the greatest saboteurs of our own lives?

I challenge you to ask the following questions:

Do you live under your means?

Do you eat foods that enhance your performance and health?

Do you exercise on a daily basis?

Do you specifically work on improving your character and values on a daily basis?

Do you focus on helping others?

Do you encourage or discourage others on a daily basis?

Do you encourage or discourage yourself to lead a healthy lifestyle?

Do you practice kindness even in the face or rudeness or insult? Or are you just kind to those who are kind to you?

There's a war going on out there and inside each of us. Recognize the battleground within yourself and you're on the road to victory.

Sometimes during my workouts while dressed in military-style attire I get comments and questions. "Where's the war?" Or "Looks like you're dressed for battle." or "Is there a war going on here?" or "Are we under attack?" My response is "Yes. There's a war going on in America."

Here are the casualties of the health war going on in the United States:

Enemy Soldiers in America		
ENEMY SOLDIER	AMERICANS KILLED	AMERICAN CASUALTIES
Heart Disease	500,000	29 million
Cancer	550,000	15 million
Stroke	150,000	6 million
Diabetes	400,000	18.2 million
Total	1,600,000	68.2 million
Totals Per Day	4,400	18 million

source: Centers for Disease Control

But who, what or where is the enemy?

What the enemy is NOT:

1. Corporate America
2. Television
3. Radio
4. Food selection at the grocery story or restaurants
5. Food manufacturers, processors and distributors
6. Advertising industry

THE REAL "ENEMY SOLDIER" IS INSIDE EACH OF US

As Walt Kelly once said, *"We have met the enemy and he is us."* In many cases, we are just like the Wildebeests that cross a crocodile infested river. Everyone else is doing it. I might as well follow along. Right? Wrong!

This reminds me of a scene I saw on Animal Planet. A river in Africa heavily infested with Crocodiles. A herd of Wildebeests approach the edge of the river and wait. You can "feel" the desire to cross mixed with anxiety and indecision. They seem to know that danger awaits them as soon as they hit the water. They know they want to reach the other side to continue their journey. Suddenly, the first few take the plunge and the feast of the crocodiles begins with the river red with Wildebeest blood.

Despite this, the rest follow. This is very similar to our situation. This all sounds so futile, you may think. How can we possibly make the change? Ours is a slow death and the enemy is not as evident and visible.

The solution is to take control one step at a time. Start focusing on what you *can* do, and the journey on the road to better health and a better life begins.

The successful warrior is the average man with laser-like focus.

- Bruce Lee

PART ONE

Ground Rules for Success

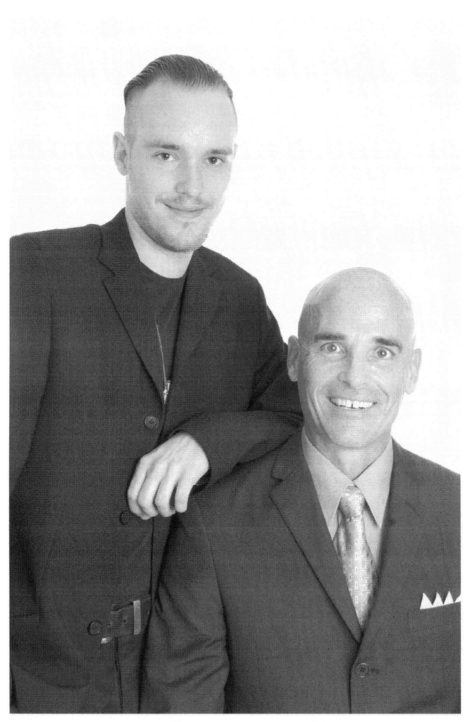

Bob Weinstein with son David

Chapter One

Core Values and Character

Change Your Character

"It is honorable to be a warrior and soldier. As with being a good soldier there are core values and character qualities that make up being a good citizen." – Lt. Col. Bob Weinstein, (ret.)

There is a reason why core values and character are discussed and presented first. Values-based living and working is a prerequisite for accomplishing a truly rewarding and enriched life. Values-based living is to be the driving force behind exercise, eating healthy and everything else we undertake in our lives. Exercise and healthy eating are not more important than a strong, values based life. Having said that, I expect you to read, absorb, think about and practice what I am about to share with you.

As you go through the core values discussed, keep in mind that there is an overriding, all-encompassing natural law that is recognized – although not always practiced! – by all cultures. That natural law or value is the Golden Rule. The Golden Rule means treat others as you would like to be treated. Use the perspective of a fair and balanced person who is truly seeking the best way to treat others in a difficult situation where any or some of the basic values seem to collide or are conflicting. Life is fluid and dynamic. The Golden Rule fulfills all of the natural laws or values. Keep this in mind on your own personal journey to improve your core values and character.

Treat every conflict situation as a special challenge to apply the Golden Rule. Where people behave in a less than honorable manner, always treat them honorably and with respect. No exceptions. Never allow bitterness and animosity towards anyone, whether it's a family member or a co-worker find a place in your heart. Bitterness is like taking poison and expecting the other person to die. Everything you say, do and think will be negatively influenced by bitterness and will be felt by others.

By the way, the Golden Rule also means treating yourself in an honorable and respectful manner. A solid character with sound core values is a major part of healthy living.

So, how will you get started? Pick up your marching orders right here and get ready to take charge of your life. It's time for some basic training.

IT DEPENDS

Is it honorable to be a warrior? Is being a soldier an honorable occupation? I asked the question and received a variety of answers. One of the responses I got was, "It depends on the soldier." Actually, the response is a good one, though with this immediate response I detected an undertone of "well, maybe not" or "necessary evil." The response "It depends on the soldier." could be applied universally as follows:

It depends on the lawyer, it depends on the doctor, it depends on the politician, it depends on the boss, it depends on the police officer, it depends on the judge, it depends on the teacher, it depends on the employee, it depends on the wife, it depends on the husband and on and on go the "it depends."

IT DEPENDS ON WHAT?

It depends. It depends. It depends. Cease Fire! Enough! Focus Soldier! It depends on what?

GET SPECIFIC AND STOP THE GENERALITIES

Let's get specific and concrete. Step smartly away from those generalities. So you want to lose weight and get in shape. I'm going to play the "It depends" game just to make a point. Pay attention! Is it honorable to lose excess weight, eat right and get and stay in shape? Well, it depends.

WHAT'S YOUR EXCUSE?

Let's take a look at the "it depends" list:

It depends on:

Time

Money

Age

Health

Education

Job

Wife

Husband

Girlfriend

Boyfriend

Children

Work schedule

Boss

I think you get the point. The point is there is no good reason or circumstance except possible medical issues.

Consequently, the response "it depends" has very little meaning.

Yes, it is honorable to be a warrior and soldier. Remember to honor our warriors. As with being a good soldier there are core values and character qualities that make up being a good citizen as well.

YOUR MARCHING ORDERS

You are now a soldier. That's right! You are a soldier on the battlefield of life. Get those combat boots on and get ready to move out! You have now been recruited into my army. In a few moments, you will receive your overall mission, "the Commander's Intent," so that when you move out smartly, you are not left in the dark as to what is expected of you. Since you may be a civilian, I don't want to make this too technical for you. We'll keep it straightforward and simple. I think you already know some basics of soldiering. This is what I expect of you, so listen up! I'm going to lay some important groundwork so that you are prepared for both peacetime and wartime operations and whatever worthy cause you may be committed to in the course of your life mission. No shortcuts here, Soldier!

NO-COST HEALTH INSURANCE – A DREAM COME TRUE

I'm about to prepare you to fight and win the health battles of life. Now, I know we usually associate the word, "health," with going to the doctor or taking prescription medication or getting health insurance. In actuality, health is the lifestyle you lead and the choices you make, good or bad.

I am going to offer you a medical insurance policy where your premiums will be made up of healthy eating, regular exercise and healthy thoughts. Save afortune and save a life – your own. These premiums will not cost you a thing. The only price will be a lifestyle change. The rewards are enormous.

MY EXPECTATIONS FOR CHANGE

GOOD ORDER AND DISCIPLINE

I expect good order and discipline. No slackers and no more excuses. Anytime you sense an excuse surfacing inside of you, I want you to shout, "Cease fire!" And if you happen to be too embarrassed to shout it out, say it or think it to yourself. Focus on what needs to be accomplished, and you will succeed in life. Yeah, I know about those obstacles, emergencies, and difficulties that from time to time will confront you as you accomplish your life mission. I want you toconstantly "see" where you want to go and which direction you want to take your life. If you do that, you won't have time to "see" the obstacles that are only there to go over, under, around or through. So chin up, straighten up that posture, and get ready to move out fearlessly, with confidence.

TAKE A STEP BACK AND GET THE BIG PICTURE

Just as an artist paints a masterpiece, you are "painting" your life with every "stroke" or decision, thought, word, deed and move that you make. Every stroke of the brush determines what the finished product will be or how it will turn out. As with an artist, everything you do or think, from day to day, year after year, is coming together to form a complete picture of your life.

Have you ever watched an artist step back from his painting to contemplate where he is and to visualize where he wants to go? Step back from your life and take a look at your "painting." Be courageous. Be creative. Be concrete. Ask yourself what realistic steps you can take to touch up your masterpiece even if it means making some changes because you recognize that you're "painting" or lifestyle is not going in the right direction. The brush of your painting is in your hand. You decide what to do with it.

YES, YOU *CAN* CHANGE

Strengthening the character is an integral part of strength training. We've heard about good and bad character. We've heard or even said, "That's the way he is" or "That's the way she is" or you've even said, "That's the way I am." We all have unique personalities and certain traits. However, character traits are all behaviors. All behaviors can be changed and modified. Please, never again say to yourself that you cannot change. If you feel that thought coming on, shout "Cease fire!" As Henry Ford once said,

"If you say you can, you can. If you say you can't, you can't."

ARMY CORE VALUES

Spend a few minutes every day assessing your behavior and interaction with others. Let's take a look at the Army core values. Whether it's at your place of work or at home, you will discover the importance of these basic values that are not only timeless but essential.

There are seven basic Army core values.

1. **Loyalty** - Bear true faith and allegiance to the U.S. Constitution, the Army and other soldiers. Be loyal to the nation and its heritage.
2. **Duty** - Fulfill your obligations. Accept responsibility for your own actions and those entrusted to your care. Find opportunities to improve yourself for the good of the group.
3. **Respect** - Rely upon the Golden Rule. How we consider others reflects upon each of us, both personally and as a professional organization.
4. **Selfless service** - Put the welfare of the nation, the Army, and your subordinates before your own. Selfless service leads to organizational teamwork and encompasses discipline, self-control and faith in the system.
5. **Honor** - Live up to all the Army values.
6. **Integrity** - Do what is right, legally and morally. Be willing to do what is right even when no one is looking. It is our "moral compass" and inner voice.

7. **Personal courage** - Develop your ability to face fear, danger, or adversity, both physical and moral courage.

Source: US Army website and respective manuals.

TRANSLATION OF ARMY CORE VALUES FOR CIVILIANS

The Army core values are timeless and universal values that have their civilian application. This is how I interpret these values for civilians.

1. **Loyalty** - Be there for your friends, family, employer, government or other organization you belong to and are a part of. Be the one who others can depend upon. I'm sure you've heard the phrase, "I've got your back." It's a great feeling when we know we have the loyal support of others. You are to be that same loyal support for others to rely on.
2. **Duty** - The same definition as used for soldiers applies to civilians as well. Accept responsibility and fulfill your obligations. Work on constantly improving yourself, especially your character. And if you should doubt that you can improve your character as you read this, shout "Cease fire!" and replace those thoughts with "I-can-do-it!" thoughts.
3. **Golden Rule** - Practice and live by the Golden Rule. Do unto others as you would have them do unto you. This, of course, requires you to be kind to yourself as well. Test your application of the Golden Rule every single day and learn from your mistakes so that you can improve and get better at practicing the Golden Rule. So how do you get better at it? The best time to practice the Golden Rule is when you would like to respond in a less-than- golden manner. Whether it's driving in traffic, grocery shopping, or speaking with a family member, friend, or foe, always practice the Golden Rule.
4. **Selfless service** - Focus on serving others in every situation, whether pleasant or unpleasant, and you will gain the most out of life. You will have better relationships, make better business decisions, and see that service to others is an essential key to strengthening your character. Another great benefit is that you will attract more people who will help and support you in your worthy endeavors.
5. **Honor** - Live up to all the values. If you're wrong, say so. It's honorable. If you may be wrong, say so. It's honorable. If someone makes a mistake and has behaved towards you in a less than honorable manner, be

honorable. Treat that person graciously. Make sure your mind, tongue, body language and attitude all express what is honorable. Fulfilling all these values is the honorable thing to do even as it relates to your health, fitness, how you eat and how you live.

6. **Integrity** - When standing at the crossroads of doing what is right or what is comfortable, do what is right. You can't imagine how integrity – or the lack thereof – will impact your physical and mental performance. Doing the right thing is a huge energy booster and will actually help strengthen your immune system. Do that daily inventory on your level of honesty and take corrective action where you notice that you've fallen short. The right attitude will always lead to honest behavior. What is right is written on our hearts so always ask yourself what is the right thing to say or do when faced with a situation or decision.

7. **Personal courage** - It takes courage to do the right thing when others may just take the low road -- or, better said, the comfortable road -- while sacrificing the right thing. That's moral courage. I'd say moral courage is what is needed to carry out the values of loyalty, duty, respect, selfless service, honor and integrity. Without courage many of these values will fall through the cracks. And if they do, just get right back up again and say to yourself, "I'll do it better next time." And keep working it like a muscle. Character values, like muscles, need to be worked on a regular basis to get and stay strong. "Use it or lose it" applies to character values as well. Seek out books that are about strengthening character. Seek out people who are on the same journey. We all need a support system.

MARCHING ORDERS – CORE VALUES AND CHARACTER

Motives matter and character matters. Don't you ever let anyone tell you or convince you that character is not important or that character cannot be changed. Improve your character and you will improve your success in the areas of health, fitness and much more.

Loyalty, duty, respect, selfless service, honor, integrity and personal courage are the character values to embrace and make a part of your life. That's an order, Soldier!

Any thought to the contrary needs to be dropped for push-ups until it surrenders!

Take one of the core values that needs some fine-tuning and work it like a muscle.

Chapter Two

War-Game Your Health

A Test for Change

"Self-deceptive thoughts are destructive and must be shot dead like an enemy that is about to take your life and the lives of others."
– Lt. Col. Bob Weinstein, (ret.)

Your next task or mission is to war-game your health. What I mean by war-gaming your health is to take inventory of where you really are in your life as it relates to health and wellness, action-plan any corrections and immediately begin implementation for change. I have devised a basic lifestyle questionnaire that will allow you to determine what areas need fine tuning and improvement. Please don't be overwhelmed or afraid. Remember that we all feel some fear when we know that some necessary lifestyle changes will be identified. Take a gradual but determined approach, and you will succeed. You are capable of accomplishing all lifestyle areas that I cover and consider essential.

My health and lifestyle questionnaire will answer the following question from the standpoint of how you lead your life and not from the standpoint of a medical examination:

What is the state of your health and how can you improve it? Please note that this question does not ask how your doctor, medical clinic, medications or health insurance will improve your health. The question deals exclusively with things that only you can do. You are going to take back control and take responsibility for your health and well-being.

You will learn:

Cause and effect of healthy and unhealthy living.

How to develop your own course of action for excellent health.

HOW AMERICANS THINK ABOUT THEIR HEALTH:

76% of Americans believe they have healthy eating habits (2004 poll conducted by Ipsos-Insight).

57% of those polled thought they were overweight.

90% of Americans know that most people are overweight,

Only 40 percent think *they* are overweight, says a phone survey of 2000 adults conducted by the Pew Research Center.

More than 60% of American adults do not get at least 30 minutes of physical activity a day and 25% of American adults aren't physically active at all.

A telephone poll of 1,072 adults conducted for Cooking Light magazine by GfK Roper Public Affairs & Media among a national sample of 1,072 adults 18 or older revealed the following:

6 percent of American adults get 30 minutes of exercise a day

22 percent exercise three to four times per week

19 percent walk or bike instead of taking more sedentary means of transportation

41 percent take the stairs whenever possible

33 percent regularly park their cars farther from their destination to work to get in extra walking

WAR-GAME YOUR HEALTH

War-gaming is a technique used to visualize the battlefield before going to battle. Several courses of action are then developed and played through to the end to assess what the probable outcome would be. This allows the commander and his staff to further refine a course or courses of action which are all focused on accomplishing the mission. Not a shot has been fired, and there is no risk, since this is really a mental exercise designed to maximize success and minimize loss of life and casualties.   This war-gaming technique can be applied to all life decisions and that is why you will apply it here.

Now, I want you to war-game your health. Put on your commander's hat and take charge. You will now develop courses of action. Excuses have no place in the analysis of a battle, whether it's a battle for better health or on the battlefield where the danger of dying or becoming a casualty is very high. Treat this analysis of your health the same way. Remember, I don't associate health with "health" insurance or visiting the doctor. I associate good health with a healthy lifestyle. As you are reading this, it may very well be happening that those snipers in the form of excuses, justifications, or even fear of some sort of change begin to surround you and take aim on your resolve. Cease fire! Fight them back! They are the enemy. They are not your friend.

THE 12 WARNING SIGNS OF HEALTH

Before we get down and dirty with the war-gaming briefing and assessment, I'd like to share with you something very inspiring that has been passed around in cyberspace. The author is unknown. The message is priceless. They are called the twelve warning signs of health.

1. Persistent presence of support network.
2. Chronic positive expectations; tendency to frame events in a constructive light.
3. Episodic peak experience.
4. Sense of spiritual involvement.
5. Increased sensitivity.
6. Tendency to adapt to changing conditions.
7. Rapid response and recovery of adrenaline system due to repeated challenges.
8. Increased appetite for physical activity.
9. Tendency to identify and communicate feelings.
10. Repeated episodes of gratitude, generosity or related emotions.
11. Compulsion to contribute to society.
12. Persistent sense of humor.
Source: unknown

Embrace and experience these warning signs of health and amazing things will happen to you.

TAKE THE HEALTH/LIFESTYLE ASSESSMENT TEST

Now it's time to do some health war-gaming. Here's a quick and simple test, which is focused on just a few of the many benchmarks of a healthy lifestyle. Answer the questions with yes or no. Your mission is to gradually but steadily move in the direction of the maximum score. If that thought starts infiltrating your mind to find the "passing" score or – as I call it – the how-can-I-just-get-by score, I think you know what to say. Cease fire!

Some of these points relate to our society and prevalence of inactivity, junk food and oversized portions and overabundance of processed foods.

	Colonel Bob's Health/Lifestyle Test	Yes	No
1.	Do you exercise at least five hours per week?	1	0
2.	Do you eat a balanced diet predominantly made up of plant-based foods that are unprocessed or minimally processed (fruits, vegetables, whole grains, nuts)?	1	0
3.	Do you eat fried foods?	0	1
4.	Do you eat meat or other animal products more than once a day?	0	1
5.	Do you regularly eat dairy products (milk, cheese, yogurt)?	0	1
6.	Do you drink water as your beverage of choice?	1	0
7.	Do you smoke?	0	1
8.	Do you drink alcohol regularly?	0	1
9.	Do you regularly spend at least 10 to 15 minutes a day of quiet time?	1	0
10.	Do you take medication, prescription or non-prescription, on a regular basis?	0	1
11.	Do you take drugs?	0	1
12.	Do you get at least six to eight hours of sleep a night?	1	0
13.	Do you spend the day thinking mostly positive thoughts?	1	0
14.	Do you work on improving your character regularly?	1	0
15.	Do you, as a rule, complain about something on a daily basis?	0	1
16.	Do you regularly worry about something?	0	1
17.	Do you take a multi-vitamin supplement?	1	0
18.	Do you take in more food and beverage than you need on a regular basis?	0	1
19.	Do you use any of these words frequently, on a daily basis? Angry, frustrated, stressed, bothers me, but, can't, don't have the time.	0	1
20.	Do you hold a grudge against anyone (family member, business associate, friend, boss, enemy, acquaintance)?	0	1
21.	Do you volunteer to help those who are less fortunate than you?	1	0

Add up your lifestyle score. If you scored 21 points, you maxed out the test and lead a very healthy lifestyle. Reward yourself with twenty push-ups! If, on the other hand, you score less than 21 points, that is a *no-go*, and you need to work on maxing the test.

MARCHING ORDERS – WAR-GAME YOUR HEALTH – A TEST FOR CHANGE

If you received zero points for any of the above questions, they now become a part of your ACTION PLAN for improvement of your life. Tackle one to three of them at a time and work them like a muscle.

CHECK FOR SELF-DECEPTION

If you gave yourself a high score or you got the maximum number of points, I want you to go back and reassess your answers. This time I want you to identify any possible sources of self-deception that may have occurred. There is this paradoxical tendency to sugar-coat the truth till it's partially or completely unrecognizable. If you happen to discover any stealthy self-deception on any of the answers to the above questions, it's time to shout, again. Go ahead. Say it. Here we go! Cease fire!

Self-deceptive thoughts are destructive and must be shot dead like an enemy who is about to take your life and the lives of others.

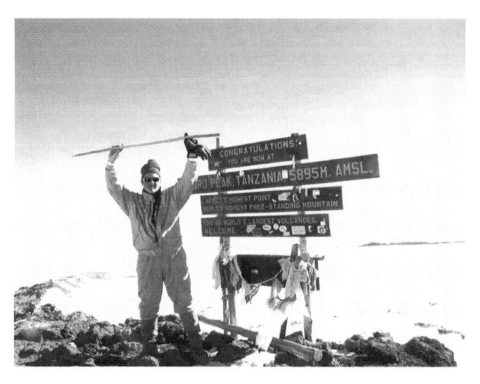

Client Albert Miniaci on the Summit of Kilimanjaro

Chapter Three

Six Keys To Permanent Weight-Loss

Change Your Weight

"It has nothing to do with eating or exercise and has everything to do with how we think." Lt. Col. Bob Weinstein, (ret.)

Since over-consumption of food combined with lack of physical activity have resulted in high numbers of Americans of all ages to be overweight, it is essential that I unlock the door to long-term weight-loss. I have identified six foundational keys to permanent weight-loss and management.

The six weight-loss keys we will cover are:

Key #1 – No more excuses
Key #2 – Talk to win
Key #3 – Think to win
Key #4 – Eat to win
Key #5 – Like how you look
Key #6 – Move

These keys leave the realm of the quick-fix society and will successfully lead to long-term weight-loss and weight management.

We all need a little body fat, so don't go trying to lose body fat till you're skin and bones and/or can't find anything to pinch. Washboard abs visible to the point of no fat may be unhealthy and may cause your immune system to suffer, making you susceptible to disease and illness.

My goal with this chapter is to help you stop yo-yo dieting and perhapsreduce any health-related suffering you may have.

OVERWEIGHT AND OBESITY EPIDEMIC IN AMERICA:

According to a study by the Centers for Disease Control, Americans are consuming more calories, on average, than they were 30 years ago—200 to 300 calories a day more. That's 73,000 to 109,500 calories per year. 3,500 calories equal one pound of fat. If these are excess calories, that translates to 21 to 31 pounds of fat in one year!

An estimated 300,000 premature deaths and more than $90 billion in healthcare costs can be attributed to inactivity and obesity.

50% of Americans are overweight, 33% are obese and as many as 40% of women and 25% of men are trying to lose weight at any given time.

Americans spend at least $30 billion a year on commercial weight-loss programs and products, and another $5 to $6 billion on fraudulent products.

Being overweight is the second leading cause of preventable death in the US.

OVERWEIGHT AND OBESITY EPIDEMIC GOES GLOBAL

Between half and two-thirds of men and women in 63 countries across five continents – not including the US – were overweight or obese in 2006.

Canada and South Africa led in the percentage of overweight people with an average BMI of 29 among both men and women in Canada and 29among South African women.

In Northern Europe, men had an average BMI of 27 and women 26.

In Southern Europe, the average BMI was 28.

In Australia BMI was 28 for men and 27.5 for women.

In Latin America the average BMI was just under 28.

A BMI of 25 is deemed overweight and greater than 30 is obese.

Source: The International Day for the Evaluation of Obesity (IDEA) study.
BMI or Body Mass Index values:

Underweight: Below 18.5
Healthy weight: 18.5 to 24.9
Overweight: 25 to 29.9
Obese: 30 or higher

SELF-DECEPTION AT WORK

90% of Americans know that most people are overweight, but only 40% think they are overweight, according to a phone survey of 2,000 adults conducted by the Pew Research Center. This self-deception stems partly from overestimating height: the average woman overestimates her height by one inch; the average man, by two inches. The study also found that the fraction of Americans who say they've dieted at some point in their lives has fallen from 57% in 1991 to 52% today.

BEWARE OF SELF-DENIAL

So a huge portion of the US population is on a diet or counting calories in one way or another. 90% of those who lose excess weight, however, gain it all back within twelve months. Why? Because of their self-talk -- or maybe I should say self-deceit.

"I'm not really overweight. I'll just lose a few pounds and that will be that." Or they say, "I'll start exercising when I lose that excess weight." What a paradox!

DIETING NEVER WORKS (LONG-TERM)

This self-denial is a fatal error and one that keeps people spending billions every year on those fake programs and products. The truth is, dieting by itself doesn't work. So let me make it clear that this chapter is really not just about weight-loss. It's about addressing the real issue: the quality of your lifestyle and how you really feel about yourself and others. How you design your life inevitably dictates the quality of your health. Every decision you make in your life has consequences, good or bad. I want to empower you to live the life that will make you truly happy and fulfilled.

The Health Colonel's weight-loss and management is not about quick fixes. I don't measure success in pounds or inches lost, or how strong you are, or how fast you can run, or how great you look.

Here's how I measure success, and you should, too:

Reduced health risk factors
Improvement in medical conditions
Improved quality of life
Improved psychological functioning
Decreased reliance on medications
Positive self-image
Regular physical activity
Healthy eating

Many of my clients make promises about what they will do, without any commitment to, or belief in, what they said. You've probably heard, or maybe even said, "Sure, I'll be there" to an invitation, and then simply didn't show up or called that day with a fabricated reason for not attending. Many people who say "I'm going to eat right and exercise regularly" or "I'm going to lose 20 pounds and keep it off" do the same thing—they just don't show up or follow through.

WEIGHT-LOSS KEY #1 – NO MORE EXCUSES

The more you do what is right in the course of your life, the more motivated and energized you become to continue on this path and to take it to the next level. It becomes fun and it changes your way of thinking for the better. - Lt. Col. Bob Weinstein, (ret.)

What you say to yourself and others has a greater impact on your life than you could ever imagine. We are creatures of habit. All our habits, both negative and positive, make up our lifestyle - how we live, both in the workplace and at home. Truth, honesty and integrity impact the quality of your life, from eating to exercise to your relationships. This is a sober fact, and here's the reason. The more you do what is right in the course of your life, the more motivated and energized you become, to continue on this path and to take it to the next level. It becomes fun and it changes your way of thinking for the better.

> *Doing the right thing begets more of doing the right thing. You actually will have more energy to do so simply by doing so.*

Living a life filled with culturally acceptable untruths is harmful to your health. OK, OK, I mean lies. But you and I know that when a fib is not serious, we tend to call it something less than a lie - an exaggeration, perhaps - or an excuse. Here are some examples:

> *"Suzy, did you do your homework last night?"*
> *"Yes, Mom. I did it while watching TV."*

Suzy didn't even crack a book. But she didn't totally lie; she did watch TV.

> *"Hey Sam, how big was that fish you caught the other day?"*
> *"Oh, man, you should have seen it. It was at least a 30-pounder."*

Yeah, right! One that weighed about 10 pounds!

> *"Marilyn, have you been going to the gym regularly like you promised?"*
> *"Well, yes, I've been going."*

Sure, she's been going, all right. Going right past it on her way to the donut shop.

You may think these are harmless examples. They are not. How we respond in so-called harmless situations is the precursor of our responses when it really does count. When we exaggerate or make excuses, we are building a habit of not telling the truth, and we are programming our own behavior so that it becomes more difficult to even tell the truth. If we continue to follow this path, we eventually end up redefining "truth," so that the truth or doing the right thing or following through with worthy goals, such as changing eating habits, losing weight or getting in shape, will lose its meaning.

THE PARADOX OF EXCUSES

We become experts in creating excuses for why we can't do what we recognize to be important. Boy, does that sound like a paradox! Imagine that! Finding and creating excuses for not doing what you have recognized to be important in your life. Just the other day, I had a conversation with a young lady. We'll call her Brenda. The conversation went like this: "Brenda, how important is your health to you, on a scale of 1 to 10, with 10 being most important?"

Brenda responded without hesitation, "My health is one of the most important things in my life. I give it 10 points."

BRENDA'S PARADOX

"Well, Brenda," I asked, "How often do you exercise each week?" She answered reluctantly, "I don't really have the time to exercise."

"Wait a minute," I said. "Let me get this straight. You just told me that your health is one of the most important things in your life, but your actions don't correspond. Explain that to me." She could not.

So what does Brenda need to do? Her words and thoughts on the importance of health don't match her actions. You see, she has made it acceptable to herself to *understand* how important her health is. Not one bit more. She sees that as enough. No action. No follow-through. Just awareness. She even had a quick excuse to keep her from taking action. As Zig Ziglar, the famous motivational speaker and author, says, *"The chief cause of failure and unhappiness is trading what you want most for what you want now."* Brenda is trading her health for a little extra time now. What a paradox!

EXCUSES REQUIRE PRACTICE AND TRAINING

A lot of training goes into making excuses, and people spend time carefully thinking of plausible ones. There are even several websites devoted to the art of making excuses. I just looked at one called "The Mother of All Excuses." You can read or submit excuses for not going to work, skipping school, speeding, running a red light, having an accident, breaking dates, missing church, and more.

Some other excuse-generating websites are The Random Excuse Generator, IShouldBeWorking.com and Sickday Excuse Generator. Here are some of the excuses I found:

SCHOOL EXCUSES

Please excuse Tommy for being absent yesterday. He had diarrhea and his boots leak.

I didn't come to school yesterday because I was feeling like I was going to be sick, but thankfully I wasn't!

DATING EXCUSES

I would love to go out with you, but I need to ask my fiancé, and I don't think he would like that very much.

I gained 5 pounds this week, and I really don't want you to see me like this.

MORE PARADOXICAL EXCUSES

Exercise excuses:

My workout clothes don't match.

My cat's depressed.

It's a bad hair day.

I don't have time to exercise.

I didn't shave my legs.

Somebody was using my treadmill.

I'm too old.

We're all going to die anyway.

EATING EXCUSES

Eating right costs too much.

I can't fit in the recommended five daily servings of fruits and vegetables.

I don't have time to eat right.

My sweet tooth rules, so I can't eat well.

I enjoy fast food too much to eat right.

It doesn't matter that I have a lousy diet, because I take a vitamin pill.

I eat too much to ever be able to eat right.

Other people in my household eat poorly, so I do, too.

We're all going to die anyway.

Cease fire! When you feel an excuse coming on, stop it in its tracks.

TAKE CHARGE

No more excuses means doing what you say you are going to do and following through with the right thing. It's about personal accountability. Excuses are a practiced form of giving up control to external circumstances or people. Taking charge of your life means focusing on what you can do - *possibilities talk*. Excuses are *impossibilities talk*. If you have recognized that weight management, healthy eating and regular exercise are priorities for you, but you practice *impossibilities talk* by programming yourself through excuses, you have made it impossible to succeed in this area. You have created a barrier or wall preventing positive change.

Have the courage to take that positive first step in the direction you have recognized is best for you. Once you have realized what is really important for your life in the long term and you are totally convinced that it is _ the right thing, pursue it like your life depended on it. Because it does. Eliminate all excuses.

BE PATIENT AND CONSISTENT

Embarking on a life of good habits doesn't have to be done in giant steps. Take it one small step at a time. Be kind to yourself and enjoy the journey. Allow for gradual change in the right _direction for your life. Have enough patience to let time take its course. Any change in your diet or lifestyle that improves your personal health, however small, is a step in the right direction.

WEIGHT-LOSS MARCHING ORDER #1 – NO MORE EXCUSES

Continue to do this

Write down one thing you will continue to do and talk about that calls for personal responsibility in what you say (Examples: Planning and accomplishing exercise every week, reducing or controlling portion sizes during all meals).

Improve this

Write down one thing you say that you don't always follow through on, something that needs improvement because you have recognized that it is important for you (Examples: eating lots of fruits and vegetables, reducing bread consumption, cutting out sweets).

Stop doing this

Finally, write down one excuse about your health that you will stop using and the positive, empowering statement you will replace it with. For instance, instead of "I'm too tired" or "I'm too busy" or "It's a bad hair day," use Possibilities Talk: "I'll make the time and schedule exercise four to six times a week to be a part of my life, and I will follow through." Put it in your weekly calendar.

Most people spend more time and energy going around problems than in trying to solve them.

- Henry Ford

WEIGHT-LOSS KEY #2 – TALK TO WIN

Discouraging and disempowering talk and self-talk will drain you of the positive emotions you need to accomplish life's many tasks, excel at work and nurture relationships. - Lt. Col. Bob Weinstein, (ret.)

What you say to others and yourself plays a key role in how successful you will be in bringing about positive change in your life. Every word of praise or kindness to others, or to yourself, actually programs you in a very positive and beneficial way.

You know eating properly and exercising are both positive. Right? How do you talk about these topics? Are you making empowering statements or disempowering ones? Are your thoughts focused on the positive or are they burdened by negative undertones? Remember that negativity is more than just the words you say!

There are emotions behind everything we say. Emotional energy is a primary source of life energy. Discouraging and disempowering talk will drain you of the positive emotions you need to accomplish life's many tasks, excel at work and nurture relationships. "Talk to win" refers to nonverbal communication as well. Walk, talk, stand and act with confidence. It will support you emotionally in the accomplishment of your worthy goals.

90% of those who lose excess weight, gain it all back within twelve months. Why? Because of their self-talk, or maybe I should say self-deceit. Let's examine the language we use about eating and exercise with Give-up vs. Take-charge talk.

GIVE-UP VERSUS TAKE-CHARGE TALK

Give-up: Should I have it?
Take-charge: Do I need it? Do I want it?

Give-up: I'll be successful once I lose those twenty pounds.
Take-charge: I am successful. I am listing and putting in my calendar what I need to do and I am implementing my goals now.

Give-up: I want it all or nothing.
Take-charge: I will take a gradual and long-term approach, one step at a time. I will do what I can do and never give up, because the cause is worthy.

Give-up: I eat when I'm stressed.
Take-charge: I eat when I'm hungry.

Give-up: I can only feel good about myself if I lose that weight.
Take-charge: I accept and like myself as I am with or without excess weight.

Give-up: Exercise means "no pain, no gain."
Take-charge: I like energetic daily living. It's fun! It's nature's Viagra.
It gives me more energy.

Give-up: The diet is in control. I have no choice.
Take-charge: I am in charge. I decide what and when to eat.

Give-up: Food is the enemy. I have to deprive myself and use willpower.
Take-charge: Food is my friend and is there for my enjoyment. I decide what I eat.

Give-up: I don't have time to exercise.
Take-charge: Exercise gives me energy so I can use my time more productively. Exercise belongs in my calendar, whether it's for 10, 20, 30 or 60 minutes. It all adds up.

Take charge and take responsibility with a winning attitude. If the cause is worthy, never, ever give up.

WEIGHT-LOSS MARCHING ORDER #2 – TALK TO WIN

Take charge

Transform something that you say that sounds like "I give up" and convert it to "I take charge." That's an order! Commit to never using that give-up-responsibility-talk again and to sticking with your new take-charge-talk.

Listen up! Don't you let those thoughts wander or start slacking on me! Stay focused and we'll get through this together.

We've covered Weight-loss Key #1 - No More Excuses and Weight-loss Key #2 - Talk to Win.

Now it's time to cover the third key, Think to Win.

No matter how bad things are, you can always make them worse. At the same time, it's often within your power to make them better.

- Randy Pausch, The Last Lecture

WEIGHT-LOSS KEY #3 – THINK TO WIN

"Set peace of mind as your highest goal and organize your entire life around it." – Brian Tracy

Your thoughts and emotions play a key role in all aspects of your health, not just in losing weight. Your mind can heal by mobilizing your body's naturalhealing powers. You have to watch how you program your thoughts and where your thoughts dwell. Where your thoughts predominantly dwell is the difference between winning and losing. This is not snake oil. If you give up hope, the battle is lost without ever firing a shot.

PLEASURE/PAIN PRINCIPLE

This step may be trickier than you think. Your subconscious is constantly trying to trick you. Even though you may completely understand that a certain behavior is the right thing to do, your subconscious starts working to get you back to where you were, where you were comfortable. This is called the pleasure/pain principle. Your subconscious is resistant to change because change is usually associated with pain. This is what was happening with Brenda when she rated her health as a 10 and yet did not devote the necessary time.

 Bad habits are the primary cause of poor health. Our mission is to replace these bad habits with healthy ones. By replacing the bad habits with good ones, you will actually enjoy the new habits as well.

I have two powerful words that I want you to use anytime you have negative, put-down, discouraging, give-up, give-in thoughts. I think you know what they are. Take a deep breath, and say it! Cease Fire!

FOCUS ON THE POSITIVE

Think positive thoughts about yourself and what is best for your health.Create a new association of pleasure when thinking about those positive changes in your exercise and eating habits, and treat yourself with kindness—like you would treat your best friend. This will replace the tendency to dwell on negative thoughts about weight-loss.

Treat your weight-loss goal like you've already achieved it

SEE IT! FEEL IT! HEAR IT! TASTE IT! EMBRACE IT!

See, hear and feel the world around you. Visualize how you want to beNOW.

Feel the benefits and rewards NOW. Listen to the sounds that are associated with it NOW. You can do this. This potential is in you. Tap into it and imagine it NOW, to experience the positive change. Knock that "T" off "CAN'T." If you say you can't, you can't. If you say you can, you can. Bring back those enormous visualization capabilities you had as a child.

TAKE INVENTORY OF YOUR THOUGHTS

Here's a self-evaluation that's easy to do and can be fun and challenging while exploring your potential. Follow your thoughts for one or two days. List your negative and positive thoughts. Listen very carefully, because we are masters at tricking ourselves. Practice awareness of what you're thinking about yourself and others. List your negative and positive thoughts.

Are you overly critical? Overly negative? Compassionate? Allowing wisdom to rule? Always asking yourself how you would like to be treated, especially if you're not treating someone else that way? Use the Golden Rule and work on making those corrections every day. Don't kick yourself. Just say to yourself, "I'll do it better next time." Take the lifestyle assessment in Chapter 2 and war-game your health. Wherever you identify a predominant focus on negativity and complaining, turn it around. Think solutions- oriented thoughts and negativity and complaining will cease. Better yet, you will feel better and accomplish more, too.

TREAT YOURSELF LIKE YOU WOULD A BEST FRIEND

From now on, look at yourself and say nice things. Imagine the best way of treating someone special in your life and think such thoughts about *you*. Smile and say, "Hey, I like myself. I have made a mistake, but I can learn from it and do better next time. I like to enjoy life. I like to relax. I like to be good to myself. I'm worth it." That's how you would treat a friend. So introduce yourself to the very best friend you'll ever have, *you*. Now treat *you* accordingly every day and every minute of your life. Be very *kind* to *you*. This will cause you to be kind to others. You will then reap more kindness in your life. Learn to forgive yourself and others and learn to move on.

As the famous motivator, Brian Tracy, says, *"Set peace of mind as your highest goal and organize your entire life around it."* Think carefully about the situations, people and settings that give you peace of mind. Learn from them.

Start taking a gradual approach, one step at a time. Does it give you peace of mind to know that you are doing things and focusing on values that enhance your health? Of course!

Always behave like a duck - keep calm and unruffled on the surface, but paddle like the devil underneath.

- Lord Barbizon

WEIGHT-LOSS MARCHING ORDER #3 – THINK TO WIN

Take charge of your thoughts and your mind. You decide where they wander and where they dwell. Your thoughts are to focus on positive things that benefit you and others. Doing so takes your eyes off of the obstacles and keeps you on track. If you fall and if you wander off track, get up, dust yourself off and continue to march.

Go Through, Over And/Or Around All Obstacles

Focus on what you want to accomplish and not on the obstacles, and you will begin to have the feeling that there are no obstacles. That's because you now have your sights on your worthy goals. If there's a wall there, you will simply approach it and immediately go to work on a way over, through or around it.

Norman Vincent Peale sums this step up best: "A positive thinker does not refuse to recognize the negative; he [or she] refuses to dwell on it. Positive thinking is a form of thought which habitually looks for the best results from the worst conditions." In other words, dwell on positive thoughts even under negative circumstances. Dwelling on positive thoughts means focusing on what you want to accomplish, not those bumps in the road, those fires to deal with or mountains to climb. There are no quick fixes for weight-loss or weight management or life. Only your determination to make positive changes can make positive changes.

These first three keys to permanent weight-loss - #1 No More Excuses, #2 Talk to Win, #3 Think to Win - make up about 80% of your success, so concentrate on them. They are performance enhancers and success multipliers. The rest of the keys are only responsible for about 20% of your success, and that is because the first three keys will drive your success (or failure).

It's time to talk about weight-loss key #4 – Eat to Win.

Most people never run far enough on their first wind to find out they've got a second.

- William James

WEIGHT-LOSS KEY #4 – EAT TO WIN

The human body burns about 12 calories per pound of body weight per day – at rest, while sitting around watching TV or performing any other sedentary activity.

Have you ever wondered why, for so many people - especially anyone older than 30 in the U.S. - weight gain seems to be a fact of life? It's because the human body is way too efficient. It doesn't take much energy to maintain the human body at rest. And, when exercising, the human body is amazingly efficient when it comes to turning food into motion.

THE OVERWEIGHT HEALTH CRISIS IN THE U.S.

There is a health crisis in the U.S. and here are some of the symptoms.

50% of Americans are overweight
33% are obese
40% of women are trying to lose weight at any given time
25% of men are trying to lose weight at any given time
Being overweight is the second leading cause of preventable death in the US.

At rest - for example, while sitting and watching television - the human body burns only about 12 calories per pound of body weight per day. That's 26 calories per kilogram. That means if you weigh 150 pounds, your body uses only about 1,800 calories per day.

1,800 CALORIES TO STAY ALIVE

Those 1,800 calories are used to do everything you need to stay alive:

They keep your heart beating and lungs breathing.
They keep your internal organs operating properly.
They keep your brain running.
They keep your body warm.

312 MILES ON A GALLON OF GAS

If you could drink gas and digest it, you would get 312 miles on a gallon of gas. At $2.90 per gallon that would be about $0.01 per mile. I don't think I need to mention this but I will anyway. Don't drink gas. It will kill you!

In motion, the human body uses energy very efficiently. For example, aperson running a marathon—which is 26 miles, or 42 km—burns only about 2,600 calories. In other words, you burn only about 100 calories per mile when you're running. Still, the body is designed to be used. If you don't exercise, your muscles will deteriorate, your arteries could clog, and your heart will have a harder time pumping enough oxygen to the body. In short, you'll age and die faster.

Did you know that if we could drink gas and the body could actually process it as food, you would get about 912 MPG while bicycling? Now, that's great gas mileage! A gallon of gas has 31,000 calories.

If you have been dieting, you may be out of touch with your body and its signals for hunger and fullness. To get back in touch, you can do several things.

EAT REGULARLY

At least every three to six hours. Include breakfast, lunch and dinner. Add a snack if your body really signals the need. If you are physically hungry, do not fill up on water or coffee – eat something. Why? It's about getting back in touch with what your body says about hunger and responding to it. It takes three to six hours to digest a balanced breakfast, so you will be hungry by lunch time. If you eat these meals and stop eating when you're full, you will ultimately eat less at the evening meal and throughout the evening. Ignoring your natural hunger signals and undereating early in the day inevitably lead to overeating - even bingeing - later

on. Eating regularly involves resetting your internal clock to a regular pattern of meals. Once you are in the habit of eating breakfast within an hour of getting up, you will soon start waking up hungry for the morning meal.

So what if you don't eat breakfast? About 50% of overweight people do not eat breakfast. Breakfast is the most important meal, so a nutritious breakfastshould not be skipped.

What about more frequent meals, say, five to six times a day? Be careful with this one. It may lead you to eating more than you should, because you could   eat only to not miss one of those six frequent meals. Eat when you are hungry and develop the habit of eating a nutritious breakfast. If you normally don't eat breakfast, ease into it by having just a little, such as half of a banana, and working your way up to a regular sized breakfast. You should eat at least three meals a day.

EAT BALANCED MEALS

The basic premise of any good diet is variety, moderation, and balance. Let's make this step really easy. Divide your plate into thirds: One third for protein(meat, seafood, poultry, and beans) and the other two thirds for vegetables, bread, potatoes and/or pastas.

"Well, instead of figuring out portions, I'm just going to get a really big or really small plate." If that helps you to adjust, that's great. Remember the focus. It's not about legal or illegal food. It's about getting back in touch with your body and responding to its real physical hunger and basic needs and what will satisfy you, while seeking out the most nutritious choices. A healthy lifestyle is one of both moderation and balance.

HIGH-OCTANE FOOD

So let's go back to dividing your plate into thirds and follow the **15/30/55 RULE**—15% protein, 30% fat and 55% carbohydrates. If a race car driver had to use food for his race car, this would be the formula for ultimate performance, as long as the ingredients overwhelmingly are unprocessed, unrefined, highly nutritious food. No race car driver is going to put low-octane fuel in his car. No human being should put low-octane food in his body. That will impact health and performance. This does not exclude once-a-week moderate amounts of sweets or desserts. More than once a week on a regular basis is too much.

PROTEIN DOES NOT JUST RUN AROUND ON TWO OR FOUR LEGS

We all have a tendency to only count the protein that comes from animal sources, and that includes dairy. We tend to disregard the protein that comes from plant sources, thereby eating too much protein. That is hard work for the kidneys and could indicate that you are either eating too much or you're not getting enough of the nutrient-rich plant products, such as fruits, vegetables, whole grains, beans and nuts.

Eat animal products no more than once a day while eating nutrient-rich, plant-based foods, and you will give your health a big boost. As a matter of fact, complete elimination of animal products while supplementing with calcium and Vitamin B-12 is extremely healthy.

15/30/55 Rule

How much food should you eat to follow the 15/30/55 guidelines? Now we're back to the topic of calories (and quantity), which doesn't necessarily mean more food. 200 calories of vegetables take up about the same amount of space as 1,000 calories of pasta! Your body will tell you how much to eat, if you "listen" carefully and closely. And if your body is still in the learning phase of "listening," a little old-fashioned, timeless, self-discipline will do the trick.

Choose Meals And Snacks That Satisfy

If you eat what you want, you will eat less in total. You need to eat enough to fill up—food that you like. But you also need to be careful to balance carbohydrates for energy—especially more complex carbs such as sweet potatoes, oatmeal or beans—with enough protein to keep you satisfied. This balance is what keeps you satisfied until it's time to eat again.

Take Your Time

Effective eating takes time. You need to find out how good it feels to sit down to a meal pleasantly hungry and to take your time with it. You will end up satisfied and able to forget about eating between mealtimes. On the other hand, don't go telling yourself you're not going to eat a meal or healthy snack if you can't eat it slowly. That would be a fatal error. Do not skip a meal if you can avoid it. Gulp it down if you can keep it down and continue to work or do whatever you are doing.

Get Enough Fiber

25 to 30 grams of fiber a day from unprocessed, close-to-nature food is a nutrient-rich diet. A fiber-rich diet helps your body deliver nutrients to its cells. If processed food and supplements are the sources of your fiber intake, you are probably not getting a sufficient amount of nutrients, which leads to an unhealthy diet. Does that mean you have to eat a can of beans a day? I think you and I know what could happen if you did that. No, eat more green and yellow-orange vegetables, citrus and yellow-orange fruits, and whole grains.

DRINK WATER

Water is one of the four basic nutrients the body needs. The other three are protein, carbohydrates and fats. Just about every process in your body depends on water. It is the most important detoxifier available to you. It helps clean you through your skin and kidneys, helps you look younger and, yes, helps you lose weight. Even mild dehydration will slow down your metabolism as much as 3%. The slower your metabolism is, the slower your weight-loss will be. You need to drink

at least eight 8-ounce glasses a day. That's right. 64 ounces a day. Depending on the weather and the types of activities, you may need more. Not iced tea, not diet soft drinks, not powdered mixes, not fruit-flavored water in a bottle. Plain old water. Now quick. Go run and get a glass of water. I know this sounds really strict. If you feel the need to add some natural fruit flavor without the calories, by all means do so. Gradually back off of the flavoring to get used to drinking plain old H_2O again.

WHAT'S IN THAT CANTEEN, SOLDIER?

During a military training exercise many decades ago, I was stopped by a drill instructor who inspected my canteen to make sure I had water in it. He unscrewed the lid and performed a sniff test. Detecting a smell other than water – no, it wasn't whiskey or gin or any other alcoholic beverage! – he poured some of the contents onto the ground.

As he saw the bright red color of my "water," he barked at me, "That's not water!"
I quickly responded, "No, Sir!"
"What's that in your canteen, Soldier?" he shouted while I stood at attention.
"Kool-Aid, Sir!"
His barking was now getting louder, "Kool-Aid? You've got to be kidding me!"
"No, Sir! Kool-Aid!"
"That'll cost ya', Soldier! You're now officially promoted to KP duty for a week."

For those civilians who don't know what KP is, it stands for Kitchen Police and entails every imaginable kitchen duty necessary to service hundreds of troops, from mopping floors to washing dishes.

I thought I could get away with a little sweet beverage in my canteen. Red Kool-Aid was not the best choice, since my lips, gums and mouth were red. A dead give-away.

So, was my drill instructor right? Was it better to drink water without the added calories? You bet he was! One of the biggest and most consistent sources of additional daily calories is through the beverages that we regularly drink. The only exception I would make would be for the high performance athlete or for long workouts in heat and humidity.

TRAINING IN HEAT AND HUMIDITY

While training or working in heat and humidity, profuse sweating leads to electrolyte depletion. Electrolytes are substances that become ions in solution and acquire the capacity to conduct electricity. The balance of electrolytes in our bodies is essential for normal functioning of our cells and our organs. Common electrolytes are sodium, potassium, chloride, and bicarbonate.

The major electrolytes are:

sodium (Na^+)
potassium (K^+)
chloride (Cl^-)
calcium (Ca^{2+})
magnesium (Mg^{2+})
bicarbonate (HCO_3^-)
phosphate (PO_4^{2-})
sulfate (SO_4^{2-})

Electrolytes are important because they are what your cells (especially nerve, heart, muscle) use to maintain voltages across their cell membranes and to carry electrical impulses (nerve impulses, muscle contractions) across themselves and to other cells. Kidneys help keep the electrolyte concentrations balanced. During a heavy workout, especially in heat and high humidity, you lose electrolytes in your sweat, particularly sodium and potassium. These electrolytes must be replaced to keep the electrolyte concentrations of your body fluids constant. Many sports drinks have sodium chloride or potassium chloride added to them.

JUICES AND FLAVORED BEVERAGES

One level teaspoon of sugar has 16 calories and 4 grams of carbohydrate. One rounded teaspoon is actually 1-1/2 level tsps and 24 calories with 6 grams of carbohydrate. Now, let's take a look at how many teaspoons of sugar are actually in the following beverages.

Orange Juice, one 8-oz. glass, fresh pressed: 112 calories (Note: most containers have 2.5 servings, resulting in 280 total calories. 8 oz. has 21 grams of sugar or 5-¼ level teaspoons of sugar. If you buy and drink the container with 2.5 servings, you are then taking in 52.2 grams of sugar, or over 13 level teaspoons of sugar.
Gatorade, 8-oz serving, 50 calories, 14 grams of sugar which translates to over 3 level teaspoons of sugar. Ever see an 8-oz bottle of Gatorade? They're usually 16 or 24-oz containers.

Soft drink such as Coke or Pepsi, 12 oz, 155 calories, 40 grams of sugar which translates to 10 level teaspoons of sugar. Look at this! That 2.5-serving container of orange juice has more sugar than a 12-oz can of soda.

Smoothie, Banana Berry from Jamba Juice, Original size (719 grams), 518 calories, 107 grams of sugar or over 26 level teaspoons of sugar. Now, that's a sugar fix!

Starbucks Caramel Frappuccino® Light Blended Coffee, Grande (16 oz), 160 calories, 21 grams of sugar and 1.5 grams of fat.

Starbucks Caramel Frappuccino® Blended Coffee, Grande (16 oz), 380 calories, 48 grams of sugar and 15 grams of fat.

Starbucks Dulce de Leche Frappuccino® Blended Crème, Grande (16 oz), 530 calories, 71 grams of sugar and 15 grams of fat (including 9 grams of saturated fat).

EAT GOOD FAT

Let's move on to another of the four nutrients the body needs, fat. A healthy diet includes fat, good fat. The secret to weight management is not avoiding fats or eating fats. It's understanding the difference between good and bad fat.

Fat from plant sources is better and healthier for you than fat from animal sources. If your fat intake is made up of saturated, hydrogenated and Trans fats, it may have a negative impact on your health. You may not feel ill. You may just feel tired or lethargic. No more than 10% of your diet should include saturated fat, which of course means that a little regular saturated fat will probably not harm you. But Trans fats, which can be found in canola oil, soy oil, corn oil, and anything called salad oil or vegetable oil, are very bad, because they are processed with high heat to make the oils stable for a longer shelf life. Read the labels carefully. New FDA standards require that the label includes information on Trans fats.

UNPROCESSED FAT FROM PLANTS IS GOOD

Focus on getting your fat from unprocessed plant sources, such as raw nuts or flax seeds that you can grind in the coffee grinder. Also, coconut, olive, peanut and sesame oils are examples of good fats as long as they are cold-pressed. Also eat lots of fatty fish, because it contains Omega-3, a fatty acid that the body can't produce on its own. Fatty fish include mackerel, lake trout, herring, sardines, salmon, and albacore tuna—even the canned, white-chunk kind.

Please be aware that there are issues with toxins in fish. Any predatory fish will generally have more poisons because it eats lots of other fish and therefore collects the toxins in its body. Non-predatory fish can also be a source of higher levels of poisons if they are farm-raised and fed fish parts as food.

You do have another excellent natural source of Omega-3 fatty acids. Omega-3s are also found in flax seeds. Just grind them up in a coffee grinder and use them for cooking, on cereals, and in salads. This is a great alternative for vegetarians and non-vegetarians. Good fats protect against aging, improve the immune system, balance hormone production, and improve brain function and vision.

SPICE IT UP

Herbs and spices are a concentrated source of antioxidants and other plant factors. And besides, they make some dishes taste better. Get creative with spices to make healthy, close-to-nature food taste very good. The eight basic spices are:

Salt
Pepper
Onion
Red pepper
Basil
Paprika
Cumin
Garlic

ARE YOU PREDATOR OR PREY?

Treat your trip to the grocery store like a hunt. You know that every hunt has prey and predator. So which are you when you grocery-shop? If you sometimes feel like prey, you're not alone. Here's a sign I saw in the ice cream department of a grocery store: "1 to 12 servings, depending on how your day went." That sign is an attempt to make you___ the prey! Don't let it happen! Explore the options, read the labels, and carefully look for whole foods that are closer to nature, unprocessed. "Unprocessed" means food that has not been manipulated or has been minimally manipulated by man. I never saw Twinkies, white bread or pasta grow on a tree; it's processed food.

Which kind of oatmeal is processed? The instant kind or the stuff you have to cook on a stove? The kind you have to cook, of course. Which are processed, canned or frozen vegetables? Canned, of course. What about sandwich meats from the deli? Most of the sandwich meats are high in chemicals and salt and are highly processed and very unhealthy. What about foods labeled organic? Don't fall for it. Organic could be processed or natural.

The food-processing industry has managed to convince most of us that we are getting nutritional value from many processed foods, but it just isn't true. What we're actually getting is chronic malnutrition.

BE CAUTIOUS WHILE GROCERY SHOPPING

Be alert when grocery shopping. Be on the hunt. You will be surprised at the discoveries you will make, and you will raise your awareness about just what is healthier for your body and what to avoid. What to avoid is easy. Stay away from junk food and munchies—which are usually high in fat, sugar and/or salt. Eliminate, or at least greatly reduce, sugar. Replace diet beverages with water. Forget those fast-food joints even exist. When dining out, take charge of the dinner table, the server, and the menu, and you will eat healthier.

When you face your fear, most of the time you will discover that it was not really such a big threat after all. We all need some form of deeply rooted, powerful motivation. It empowers us to overcome obstacles so we can live our dreams.

- Bob Proctor

WEIGHT-LOSS MARCHING ORDER #4 – EAT TO WIN

Eat close-to-nature

The less food is manipulated by man, the healthier it is. Eat predominantly plant-based foods, because that is where the vast majority of nutrients can be found that will help the body live disease-free, have more energy, fight off illness, and actually feel better.

15/30/55 rule

Remember the rule of thumb: 15/30/55. Approx. 15% protein, 30% fat and 55% carbohydrates. Remember to count the plant-based protein. Also, test yourself for two to three typical days. Write down everything you eat and drink including all snacks, beverages and vitamin pills. Now calculate the calories and approximate the percentages of protein, fat and carbs. You may be surprised at the quantity (= calories) and percentages of protein, fat and carbs. Think about how you will adjust and, if necessary, make those changes and adjustments.

Avoid those low-carb or high protein diets

Stay away from those diets of low carbs or high protein or any of these other fancy ideas to get you away from healthy eating habits that are long-term.

Balance quantity and quality

Remember that your primary eating issues are quantity and quality. Your mission is to keep an eye on both. Reduce the quantity, if necessary, and increase the quality of food you are eating. Just reducing your quantity or manipulating the 15/30/55 rule will not result in better health. Soldier, you've got decisions to make. Now make them and move out smartly. If you feel that urge to cry or complain, cease fire! All right, a little crying is allowed. Get over it, move on and focus on what you want to accomplish. Now go out into your backyard and start burying those bad habits, one at a time. If the crying starts to linger longer than five minutes, go to my website, NoMoreCryBabies.com.

You can accomplish anything in life, provided that you do not mind who gets the credit.

- Henry Ford

WEIGHT-LOSS KEY #5 – LIKE HOW YOU LOOK

Let's move on with our Offensive Weight-loss and Management Operations. No defensive posture here. Offensive means take the initiative and take charge of the battlefield. Key #5 to unlock your own lifestyle based weight-loss/management program is to like how you look no matter how you look.

CAN YOU MORPH INTO A DIFFERENT BODY TYPE?

Did you know that there are three different body types? All of us fit into one of these types, or we may have elements of several. They are:

Endomorph is a heavy body with a soft and rounded shape.
Mesomorph is a well-developed, muscular body.
Ectomorph is a long and lean body.

Bill Clinton, John Goodman, and Roseanne Barr are endomorphs.
Arnold Schwarzenegger, Daryl Hannah, and Kevin Costner are mesomorphs.
Mia Farrow, Anthony Per kins, and Fred Astaire are ectomorphs.

DOES IT MATTER WHAT BODY TYPE YOU ARE?

Which are you? It doesn't really matter. Whatever your body type is, you can't change it. What is important to remember is that regardless of your body type, you can be healthy by eating right and exercising regularly. *An important truth to remember for all body types is that regular exercise and healthy eating will make you look better and give you more energy.* If you look better and have more energy and you allow it to shine, others will notice, too. This is extremely important because of the unrealistic "ideal" body that is perpetuated in the media. I can assure you that there are people with these bodies who are not healthy. I also know people who have a little excess extra body fat who are very healthy because of the quality of food they eat and the active lifestyles they lead.

HERE'S WHAT YOU CAN CHANGE

What you can change is how you feel about how you look. Your feelings about your looks closely tie in with how you feel about yourself. Are you really going to begin to like yourself once you achieve that ideal weight and appearance? What if you never achieve it? Does that mean that you will not accept and like yourself as much? If your thoughts have led you to believe that you first must achieve that ideal weight before you can really be satisfied or like yourself, you are in for a rude awakening. You would not treat a friend like that, because you know the true worth of a friend is not their appearance or their state of health. You won't find happiness like that, and you will therefore probably have greater difficulty accomplishing some of your life goals because you will have robbed yourself of your greatest motivator. That's you!

WEIGHT-LOSS MARCHING ORDER #5 – LIKE HOW YOU LOOK

Soldier! Listen up! You are to like and respect yourself every single day! That's an order! If you are even thinking otherwise, CEASE FIRE! That means respectful thoughts and actions all the time. Never talk down to yourself or say demeaning things to yourself or to others about yourself. Treat yourself like you would a very best friend. Value who you are, and you will enhance your daily task performance, and your successful weight management will be within your reach. Now, there is a side benefit to this approach. You will have a lot more fun and enjoyment with life and you will enjoy being around YOU. There is another side benefit. Others will enjoy being around you much more and you will attract like-minded people into your life.

It's good to have money and the things money can buy, but it's good, too, to check up once in a while and make sure you haven't lost the things money can't buy.

- George Horace Lormier

WEIGHT-LOSS KEY #6 – MOVE!

Regular exercise is the best health insurance premium, and it doesn't have to cost a thing. In fact, it may even save you a significant amount of money that you would have spent on illnesses, lost workdays and prescription medications. -Lt. Col. Bob Weinstein, USAR (ret.)

The final key to successful weight-loss and weight management requires you to move that body.

DEVELOP A PHILOSOPHY OF MOVEMENT

Develop a philosophy of movement in your life. Incorporate as much exercise and movement into your daily life as reasonably possible. Seek out activities-based things to do with your free time.

REGULAR MOVEMENT AND EXERCISE HAVE MANY BENEFITS

Exercise helps control your weight because it helps burn calories.
Exercise strengthens your body and makes it more fit and resilient.
Exercise builds muscle, which will allow your body to burn even more calories at rest.
Exercise strengthens your immune system.
Exercise promotes healing and tissue regeneration.
Exercise promotes stress management.
Exercise helps keep your heart healthy.
Exercise promotes psychological wellness.

MOVEMENT PROMOTES FAT LOSS AND MUSCLE GAIN

Weight-loss <u>without exercising</u> will result in only 3/4-pound of fat loss and 1/4-pound of muscle loss for every pound lost. Weight-loss <u>with an exercise program</u> will result in 1 ¼-pounds of fat loss and a ¼-pound gain in muscle mass for every pound lost. This is based on a safe weight-loss program of 1 to 2 pounds per week.

EXERCISE STRENGTHENS YOUR IMMUNE SYSTEM

Exercise and movement actually promote the strengthening of your immune system. Your lymphatic system plays an important role in the strength of your immune system. The lymphatic system collaborates with white blood cells in lymph nodes to protect the body from being infected by cancer cells, fungi, viruses or bacteria. There is no pump – like the heart – to pump lymphatic fluid through the system, so exercise supports the movement of lymphatic fluid and the functioning of the lymphatic system. Conversely, a sedentary lifestyle may weaken your immune system.

Find a type or types of exercises that you enjoy and do it every day for a minimum of 30 minutes. It might be walking, running with your dog, dancing, riding a stationary bike while watching TV or reading, or even cutting the grass. All movement/exercise is cumulative. That means every 10, 15, 20, 30, 40 and 60 minute time period for exercise/movement adds up to a cumulative health benefit. Every minute spent watching TV will accumulate into hours, days, weeks, months and years of being sedentary.

Don't like to exercise? Tough! Cease fire! You are hereby ordered to like exercise. Spend every morning and evening in front of the mirror expressing your fondness of exercise and how you can hardly wait to move and exercise. This is not a joke. Not liking exercise may kill you before your time or cause you to come down with a disease or incapacitation that will not be fun.

TAKE THE STAIRS

Instead of taking the elevator, take the stairs. Park farther away from stores when you go to the mall. Put a set of weights at your desk and use them three or four times during the day as you think or talk on the phone. Walk whenever you can, not whenever you have to. Walking is an ideal and natural form of exercise. It's free, it's easy, and it's convenient. How about a walking meeting, where appropriate? It tones muscles, improves fitness, helps with circulation, aids breathing, helps reduce stress and tension, and helps you lose weight and keep it off.

WALKING IS NOT ENOUGH

Please keep in mind that I am not suggesting that you can obtain complete body fitness and health simply by walking. That is not true. That skeletal structure is held up by a whole array of muscles that are not just in your legs. To keep your skeletal structure, connective tissue and nerves from being overburdened, resulting in conditions such as back pain, knee issues or issues with other body parts, exercise your complete body. You don't have to be an athlete to do that, as you will soon discover when following my guidance found in the section on exercise.

Post these orders next to your bathroom mirror, in your foot locker, your wall locker, your closet, your car and in the office. Recite it, sleep it, sing it, pray it and work it. Tell your girlfriend, boyfriend, husband, wife and anyone else you feel like telling. Stir up some positive, goal-oriented energy.

Everything comes to him who hustles while he waits.

- Thomas Edison

WEIGHT-LOSS MARCHING ORDERS
SIX KEYS TO PERMANENT WEIGHT-LOSS

Order #1 – No More Excuses – Eliminate all excuses

Do what you say you're going to do. Not following through is a roadblock to permanent weight-loss and weight management.

Order #2 – Talk to Win – Talk about goals, not obstacles

Program yourself with positive, take-charge and take-personal responsibility talk, NOT talk that focuses on external, "out-of-your-control" circumstances or people.

Order #3 – Think to Win – Dwell on the positive (= goals to accomplish), not the negative (= obstacles to overcome)

Norman Vincent Peale sums this step up best by saying, "A positive thinker does not refuse to recognize the negative, he [or she] refuses to dwell on it. Positive thinking is a form of thought which habitually looks for the best results from the worst conditions." In other words, dwell on positive thoughts even under negative circumstances. There are no quick fixes for weight-loss or weight management or life. Only your determination to make positive changes can make positive changes. Take command of your mind and your thoughts, and you will succeed.

Order #4 – Eat to Win – Balance quantity and quality of food

Watch the quantity and the quality of the foods you eat. Choose healthy food that you enjoy. Eat regularly. Eat balanced meals and eat healthful snacks that satisfy. Eat fiber-rich, predominantly plant-based foods that are minimally manipulated by man (unprocessed). Drink lots of water. Avoid fast food and junk food. Take charge of the grocery store and the dining table. Take a multi-vitamin without any thought that you will be getting health from a pill. The vitamin pill – or any other pill, supplement or powder – is no replacement for healthful, close-to-nature food.

Order #5 – Like how you look

Go look in the mirror, smile, and say words of praise and encouragement. You ARE your own best friend. Treat yourself that way, and then treat others the same.

Order #6 – Move

Physical fitness and weight management require a lifelong commitment of time and effort. Exercise must become one of those things that you do without question. Like bathing and brushing your teeth, once is not enough.

Chapter Four

Myths and Propaganda

Change Your Focus

"There are enemy soldiers on American soil. The names of these soldiers are Heart Disease, Cancer and Stroke. They are killing over 3,000 Americans a day." - Lt. Col. Bob Weinstein, USAR (ret.)

THE TRUTH IS OUT THERE

As a soldier, you will identify and neutralize the myths, lies, propaganda and disinformation disseminated by the enemy about eating and exercise. Become a model soldier of healthy living such that everything you do and say will be a guiding light for others and ultimately result in saving other lives by inspiring others to make those healthy lifestyle changes.

KNOW THE ENEMY

There are other similar enemy soldiers who kill and maim Americans every day. Why are these enemy soldiers so successful in killing so many Americans? Do you think the deaths in Iraq have killed a lot of Americans? Think again. That's no comparison to the hundreds of thousands that die needlessly every year at the hands of these enemy soldiers in the form of diseases that attack the health of Americans right on our own soil.

What is their strategy? How do they operate? What is their mission? Just how do they get into our minds? I will tell you how. They have outstanding PSYOPS

(Psychological Operations) to manipulate your mind into thinking a certain way about eating and exercise. Their mission is to constantly offer up pseudo-fixes and partial truths that keep Americans focused on short term "solutions" that are not solutions at all. Their mission is to sabotage our making the long-term, fundamental lifestyle changes that will result in a longer, healthier life. These enemy soldiers have been effective in playing on our basic cultural desire for quick gratification. These enemy soldiers are responsible for Americans spending billions of dollars on health care, medication, and various quick cosmetic fixes.

Enemy Soldiers in America

ENEMY SOLDIER	AMERICANS KILLED	AMERICAN CASUALTIES
Heart Disease	500,000	29 million
Cancer	550,000	15 million
Stroke	150,000	6 million
Diabetes	400,000	18.2 million
Total	1,600,000	68.2 million
Totals Per Day	4,400	18 million

source: Centers for Disease Control

IT'S TIME TO FIGHT BACK!

Follow me into the briefing room. After we knock out a few push-ups, I will brief you on enemy PSYOPS. This is one of those few times when you will hear me say, "Have a seat and relax." Listen up! What you're about to hear will save American lives, so pay attention. No slacking here! You are to take what you hear and learn today out into the world, act on it, and share it with others. All Americans need to know the enemy's tactics. That is the first step in adjusting mentally to defend ourselves in the war on our minds that leads to premature death and needless suffering.

These enemy myths and lies covered here are not the only ones. There are more, many more. The enemy does not sleep.

This will be a two-part briefing. One part will cover exercise myths. The other will cover eating myths. Let's get right down to business. Break out those note pads and take notes. Next week, you will brief me on enemy PSYOPS. I want to make sure you are prepared to spread the word and implement the necessary changes in your life, starting today. Good old-fashion Cold-War-era friendly-forces intel has busted these myths, lies and disinformation.

EXERCISE MYTHS

Exercise MYTH # 1: The best time to exercise is in the morning, because it jump-starts your metabolism.
The TRUTH: Exercise anywhere, anytime.
The best time to exercise is the time that fits your schedule. That can be morning, noon or nighttime. The enemy wants to rob you of any thought of flexibility so that you just surrender and don't exercise enough. Morning exercise will expedite the wake-up process, and you will feel energized. Mid-day exercise will energize and refresh you and help you overcome that afternoon grogginess. Night-time exercise is an amazing stress-management tool that will get that blood circulation back up so you're really infused with the energy to enjoy the evening much more. Any morning versus evening metabolism difference is insignificant compared to the overall benefit of exercising. It's propaganda from the enemy. This myth is busted.

Exercise MYTH # 2: If you don't exercise, muscle will turn into fat.
The TRUTH: Muscle does not and cannot turn to fat.
What a bunch of hogwash! The Wizard of Oz may be able to turn muscle into fat, but that's a fairytale, and the Tooth Fairy will not be able to help you on this one! Snap out of it, Soldier! Fat cannot and does not turn to muscle, and muscle cannot and does not turn to fat! If you even think this thought again, CEASEFIRE! Here's what does happen. You burn off fat and build muscle OR you lose muscle and gain fat. Get that other propaganda out of your head!

Exercise MYTH #3: Running a mile burns more calories than walking a mile.
The TRUTH: Both running and walking a mile burn the same amount of calories.
We called in our mathematicians for this one. They looked at us with a grin and said, "Give us something challenging. This is a no-brainer." Running one mile and walking one mile both burn 100 calories. Walking a mile takes longer

and therefore results in a burn of the same amount of calories. So why run? Because it works that cardio and, if you are looking for a calorie burn, running will burn more calories in less time than walking. Ask a mathematician. It's true.

Exercise MYTH #4: You must exercise continuously for 30 to 40 minutes to benefit your heart.

The TRUTH: Every bit of exercise adds to a heart benefit.

The enemy wants you to subscribe to the self-defeating All-or-Nothing Principle. The All-or-Nothing Principle: "If I can't exercise continuously for 30 to 40 minutes, I'm not going to do it at all." We have been created to do what we CAN do. Research supports the fact that every bit of exercise accumulates to an overall health benefit. Conversely, every bit of sedentary lifestyle accumulates to damage your health and your heart.

Exercise MYTH #5: A good sweat results in extra weight-loss.

The TRUTH: A good sweat is a good sweat.

I'll tell you what a good sweat is! It's a good sweat! A good sweat results in extra water loss, not fat weight-loss. Need I say more?

Exercise MYTH #6: If you are injured, you should not work out at all, in order to allow your injury to heal.

The TRUTH: Movement promotes healing.

My reliable agents in the field have uncovered a couple of sources of this myth. It's possible that liability concerns of the medical community may play a role in the propagation of this misinformation. The truth: Movement promotes healing as long as it is done safely and under the guidance of your physician. Now, here's a big test question for you. Why is physical therapy prescribed for injuries? Yeah, I know. I already gave you the answer: Movement promotes healing and the regeneration of tissue.

Exercise MYTH #7: Focusing on abdominal exercises will help me lose that belly fat.

The TRUTH: This inspired me to get poetic.

You can crunch all day.

You can crunch all night.

You can crunch at bedtime and by the moonlight.

You can crunch it up.

You can crunch it down.

There ain't no way you'll lose a pound.

No! Abdominal exercises do not target belly fat loss. Don't believe those gadget commercials and, by the way, there is no Tooth Fairy.

Exercise MYTH #8: Stretching before exercise is essential to prevent injury.
The TRUTH: There is no conclusive evidence that stretching prevents injury.

This myth is designed by the enemy to keep you from getting down to business and focusing on your cardio and strength training. Too much emphasis on stretching! The cardio benefit of stretching is almost zero. There is no conclusive evidence that stretching is essential to prevent injury. In fact, there are studies that suggest that stretching actually increases the muscles' susceptibility to injury, which – according to the studies – causes the muscle fibers to lengthen and destabilize the muscle during strength training. Mild stretching should not really be a problem. My recommendation: Warm up the body before stretching, or perform mild stretches until warmed up. Another option is to briefly stretch between sets.

Exercise MYTH #9: Never eat before a workout.
The TRUTH: Eat before your workout.

The enemy would like Americans to run out of energy and get weak. Now, if someone said to you, "We're going take a drive. Make sure you don't get gas," I think I can visualize that look of astonishment on your face! Food is fuel, and you need it for your workout. But don't overeat. If you have an evening workout, make sure that lunch is not the last meal you had. And if you don't have time to get a decent meal, eat a banana, a sports shake or an energy bar. There is no excuse for not getting some good-quality nourishment in preparation for a good- quality workout.

Exercise MYTH #10: Strength training with weights will make women bulk up.
The TRUTH: No! Strength training will not bulk women up.

The enemy wants to keep our women weak. Don't let it happen! Ladies, you will not bulk up with strength training. Most women's bodies do not produce enough testosterone to become bulky like those big guys on TV. Proper strength training will enhance your appearance and strength. And if you're still concerned, just concentrate on doing high reps. That strategy is very healthy for your muscles because you will also be increasing your muscle endurance and not just yourmuscle strength.

Exercise MYTH #11: You should only start strength training after losing excess weight.
The TRUTH: Strength training is great for weight-loss.
Here we go again. The longer the enemy can delay an American getting on an exercise program, the greater the chances of defeat, and another healthy lifestyle will be shot down by a myth before it even takes off. Movement isalways healthy as long as you   are not hurting yourself. Of course, in the beginning, exercise may very well hurt your feelings. If you feel that coming on, just go to my website NoMoreCryBabies.com. Strength training is a definite plus when you're in the process of losing excess weight. Cardio is also essential. Just follow that principle of doing what you can do, and don't forget to constantly say to yourself and others how much fun you are having.

Exercise MYTH #12: If you don't exercise hard and often, it's a waste of time.
The TRUTH: All exercise benefits your health.
The human body was created for movement and not a sedentary lifestyle. Every bit of exercise you can integrate into your daily life will enhance yourhealth and wellbeing. It is a myth that you must exercise hard and often to reap any health benefits. Eat right; exercise regularly; think predominantly positivethoughts; focus on those worthy life goals; focus on leaving your mark on this earth by serving others and benefiting your fellow man and woman. That's arecipe for a healthy life.

Exercise MYTH #13: You will burn more fat if you exercise longer andkeep your heart rate in the "fat burning" range.
The TRUTH: You will burn more fat when you increase the intensity.

It's time for math class, again. Yes, it's true that the *percentage* of fat you are burning with a low-intensity workout is higher than a more intense workout with a heightened heart rate. But here's the fatal math error. With a low-intensityworkout, you are burning fewer calories. With a high-intensity workout, you are burning, overall, more calories and are therefore also burning more fat, eventhough   the *percentage*   of fat burn is decreased. This means that all those treadmills with those fat burn indicators are not only robbing you of a calorieburn, but are also robbing you of a good cardio and strength training workout.

Forget those gadgets that measure your heart rate, and get back in touch with your body by using what is called perceived exertion. You can tell whether your workout is light, medium, hard, very hard, or brutal. Use that as a gauge. And remember: You want to get your heart rate up, to improve your cardiovascular condition. Otherwise, those disease-related enemy soldiers will be knocking at your door.

Exercise MYTH #14: You must stay away from strength training while trying to lose weight, since it will cause you to bulk up.

The TRUTH: All exercise, both cardio and strength training, is essential during a weight-loss program.

This one may tie in with the other myth that fat can turn to muscle. All exercise, both cardio and strength training, is essential during a weight-loss program. If you don't perform strength training, your body will begin practicing cannibalism. And guess whose muscle mass your body will eat? Your own! That's not science fiction. If you are not using and maintaining your muscle, you will lose it. Also, your metabolism will slow down even more, and your health will suffer.

Exercise MYTH #15: Stress speeds up the metabolism and burns more fat.

The TRUTH: Stress causes the body to burn fat slower and may result in increased fat retention.

Exercise MYTH #16: Jogging and running will make a woman's breasts sag.

The TRUTH: This is not a myth! Jogging and running will make a woman's breasts sag, if she doesn't wear proper support.

Wear a sports bra and don't even think of eliminating excellent cardio from your workout. Walking is for people who can't run, and I hope you're not in that category. If you don't wear a good sports bra, exercising can make your breasts sag more quickly, says Peter Bruno, M.D., an internist in New York City. High-impact activities, particularly jogging or aerobics, can stress your Cooper's ligaments, the connective tissue that keeps breasts firm. According to the American Council on Exercise, compression bras work best for smaller-busted women. The more well-endowed (typically a C cup or larger) should opt for an "encapsulation" bra that supports each breast separately. Replace workout bras every six months to a year.

Exercise MYTH #17: I can't lose weight because it's in my genes.

The TRUTH: No! Your genes do not have the last word. Eating right and exercising regularly will have a positive impact on your weight regardless of your genes. Lack of exercise and bad eating habits will have a negative impact on your health regardless of your genes.

You have no influence over your genes and, in some cases, there is a propensity for weight gain that is in the genes. But wait. The truth is exercise and healthy eating will have a positive impact on you regardless of your genes. This means that if you have the propensity to gain weight or get certain diseases, exercise and eating right will still reduce the impact.

Your lifestyle choice could have a negative impact on the development of your genes for future family generations. There is new evidence for what is called environmental inheritance, a radical theory of transgenerational genetic adaptation proposed by Professor Marcus Pembrey of the Institute of Child Health, University College of London in the mid 1990's. Simply put, your lifestyle of poor food choices or overeating or not exercising could lead future family generations to have a propensity for being overweight or having certain diseases or even smoking. The good news is that your healthy lifestyle may have a positive impact on the development of your genes for future generations.

EATING MYTHS

Eating MYTH #1: Eating fat is bad for you.

The TRUTH: Eat fat, Soldier! It's good for you. Just don't eat too much, and stay away from bad fat.

If you want to be healthy, you must have body fat, and you must eat fat. Don't eat too much, and make sure that the fat you eat is the good stuff. Eliminate the bad fats first. Trans fats and hydrogenated fats are bad news for the body. Stay away from them. Trans fats and hydrogenated fats are almost exclusively found in processed foods. Read the labels and you will quickly learn about the sources of these bad fats. Saturated fats can also be a source of artery-clogging and cholesterol-increasing fats. So where do you get those good fats? You get them from plant products (plant-based oils and nuts). Your best bet is to look for plant- based fats that contain predominantly monounsaturated fats and a lesser amount of polyunsaturated fats. Olive oil fits this description. No more than 30 % of your daily caloric intake should be made up of fat (example: one tablespoon of olive oil has 120 calories). Some athletes, like professional soccer players, actually consciously increase their fat intake to as high as 40% due to special athletic needs.

Let's take a quick look at what fat is used for in the body:

Stores energy.

Gives shape to your body.

Serves as a protective cushion to your skin.

Insulates the body to reduce heat loss.

Is a part of every cell membrane in the body.

Is essential to brain and nerve cells function.

Serves as a protective cushion around your internal organs.

Is an integral part of many hormones and other biochemicals, such as Vitamin D.

Eating MYTH #2: The best way to lose weight is to cut back on the calories.
The TRUTH: Exercising and eating right are the best ways to lose excess weight.
The best weight-loss is one where you watch the quantity and quality of food you eat and exercise regularly. If you just reduce calories, especially without exercising, your metabolism will slow down to compensate for the reduction, and your weight-loss strategy is out the window. (See the chapter on "Six Keys to Permanent Weight-loss").

Increased stress can even cause your body to store more fat. That's right. Your body has a protective mechanism when it's stressed by dieting. Merely cutting back on calories without eating healthy or exercising will cause you to lose   good, lean,   muscle   mass. This means that your body has practiced cannibalism on itself and is "eating" your flesh. As you can see, you will actually create a whole array of health issues if you listen to the enemy on this one.

Eating MYTH #3: You can eat as much as you want, if you are eating healthy foods.
The TRUTH: No! Even if you are healthy and exercise regularly, overeating healthy food choices lead to poor performance and reduced energy.
After trampling through all the other land mines (= myths) above, this should be an easy one for you. This myth focuses on the quality of food while disregarding the quantity. Truly healthy eating focuses both on the quantity and quality of food.

Eating MYTH #4: You can eat whatever you want, if you work out regularly.

The TRUTH: No! Unhealthy food choices reduce energy and physicaland mental performance.

Would you ever hear a race-car driver say, "I'm going to put low-octane fuel in that gas tank. After all, this car gets worked regularly." Performance andenergy would suffer and races would be lost. It is no different with the human body. Put low-octane fuel (= unhealthy food choices) in your body, and yourperformance will suffer. You will have less energy and more health issues. Poor food choices will impact your mood, compromise your immune system, and get your hormones out of whack. Need I say more? Occasional indulgence in foodand drink, even if it may be "low-octane fuel," will probably not negatively impact your overall health. Occasional means no more than once a week.

Eating MYTH #5: Eating late at night will cause you to gain extra weight.

The TRUTH: Eating a regular meal after 8:00 PM does not cause weight gain.

If you are hungry and are considering missing a meal because it's late, by all means, eat something. Weight gain is caused by eating too much and/or not exercising regularly. We all do not have the same schedules, so we have to design our own eating plans. Eat at least three times a day with one or two (unprocessed) healthy snacks, if necessary. We generally want to avoid eating less than an hour before bed only to prevent digestive sleep interruptions, which may result in some very interesting dreams.

Eating MYTH #6: Skipping meals is a good strategy to cut back on calories and lose weight.

The TRUTH: Skipping meals is a one-way ticket to weight gain.

Intentionally skipping meals is the fastest way to gain weight and possibly get sick. Your body is smarter than you are and will protest your skipping a meal by slowing that metabolism down so that you won't lose one single pound of fat.

Eating MYTH #7: Eating less than 1200 calories will speed up your weight-loss.

The TRUTH: Here we go again. This is a myth and will slow your metabolism making you more susceptible to weight gain. See our intel on Eating MYTH #2.

Eating MYTH #8: Salads are the best and healthiest way to eat when eating out.
The TRUTH: Leafy green stuff is not enough.

I need to send some of my troops to inspect the salad bar, though I'll bet I can guess what they'll find. They'll report that healthy-sounding salad bar has been fattened up with animal-source toppings (bacon bits and cheese shavings), other animal products (sweetened yogurt and a side of cottage cheese), and salted nuts. There is fruit drenched in sugary syrup. There may be Jell-O, which is low in fat but is a refined-sugar ammo dump. If there is an otherwise nice potato or egg salad, it is booby-trapped with an extra dose of fat in the mayo and cream cheese that's probably not that good for you unless you exercise true self-discipline and just take a taste of each or, better yet, pass them by completely.

Finally we come to the dressings. If you stick to vinegar and olive oil (Watch the quantity!) you've got a great dressing choice. The creamy dressings are the absolute killers. You will need to read the labels on the others, but I'm pretty certain you're going to find all kinds of chemicals and they will try to play with your mind by offering up labels that say "low-cal", "low-carb", "low-fat", "low- sugar" and/or "sugar-free."

Make sure you go easy on the iceberg lettuce; it's extremely low in nutrients. Exclude the corn, or spice up your salad with just a little. The optimal high-octane salad has a multitude of vegetable colors and could be sweetened optionally with fresh fruit or raisins. Add some whole grains on the side and a baked white or sweet potato, and you've got yourself a healthy salad which has complex carbs, protein and good fat (olive oil).

Eating MYTH #9: Carbohydrates are fattening and should be limited when you are on a weight-loss program.
The TRUTH: Carbs are essential for health, energy and performance.

Whatever you eat - carbs, protein and fat - will turn to fat if your intake of calories is greater than your expenditure. It's like money in the bank, except that your bank is the storage of fat (usually in unfortunate places). Choosing high-octane, close-to-nature (unprocessed) plant-based foods, comprised of approximately 55 % carbohydrates, 15 % protein and 30 % fats, is the high-performance formula for healthy eating. I'm sure some of you are looking at the 55% carbs and gasping because you have been indoctrinated by all that diet propaganda. Remember, 55 is a percentage of your food intake, not the quantity. Reduce the quantity and that 55 % carbs is a smaller portion. Your body predominantly needs carbs for energy and brain performance. Any good mathematician will confirm this.

Eating MYTH #10: Eating foods designated as "low fat" or "no fat" or "fat free" means no calories.

The TRUTH: These are the deceptive ways to offer up other calories or sweetener substitutes.

It's a trick! It's the old Trojan Horse, so don't fall for it! Fat is a huge flavor source. Take away the fat and you need to "sweeten the pot" with something else. That could be sugar or a chemical in a sugar disguise (artificial sweetener). Our level of sweetness desired is mostly due to a psychological dependence. If you continue to use a sugar substitute, you have no opportunity to lower your threshold of sweetness perception. You will continue to desire the heightenedlevel of sweetness. That is also the work of the enemy.

Eating MYTH #11: High-protein/low-carb diets are the healthy way to lose weight and to eat on a regular basis.

The TRUTH: Low-carb diets kill performance, energy and health.

I once had a client who was in pilot training for a commercial airline. The instructor began one lecture by asking the pilots, "Who is on a low-carb diet?" About ten hands went up, including the hand of my client. Speaking directly to those on the diet, the instructor gave the following orders: "From this day forward you are not on a low-carb diet. Carbohydrates are needed for alertness and brain performance, and we can't have pilots that aren't alert or are lacking the necessary brain performance." It gets worse. If you are eating a high-protein, low-carb diet, you are eating less plant-based foods. Plant-based foods contain more nutrients than the animal protein foods. The quality of foods is dictated by the proper mix of carbs, protein and fats. High protein also means more work for your kidneys. This diet does not focus on health.

Eating MYTH #12: Fast foods are always an unhealthy choice, and should not be eaten at all.

The TRUTH: Infrequent indulgence will probably not hurt.

I'm sure you've taken some multiple-choice tests in the past. The word that should jump out at you in the myth statement is "always." In fact, there are some healthy choices at fast food restaurants and lots of unhealthy ones. And if you happen to indulge in an infrequent hamburger or shake or fries, as they say in

German "Das macht die Suppe nicht heiss!" Translation: "That doesn't make the soup hot!" Infrequent indulgence will not have a significant negative impact on your health as long as you are otherwise eating healthy and exercising regularly.

Eating MYTH #13: You must eat "complete-chain protein" foods from animal products in order to get the right protein.

The TRUTH: By eating a variety of plant-based products, you can get all your essential amino acids to make sure you are getting the protein you need.

Here you have two myths wrapped into one. You don't need any animal products to get the protein amino acids your body needs. You can, for example, eat rice and beans to get the essential protein amino acids your body needs. You can eat the rice with one meal and the beans at another and your body will still process the protein. Your essential amino acids can be found in plant proteins and they do not need to be combined. Some marketing campaigns for protein supplements, especially directed towards body builders, are using this label of "complete protein" to side-track your diet towards their supplements. For more info on this topic, go to Wikipedia at en.wikipedia.org/wiki/Branched-chain_amino_acids.

MYTH BUSTING MARCHING ORDERS – MYTHS AND PROPAGANDA

During the Cold War, propaganda was the name of the game, whether in print, on the radio, or on television. If you happened to live in one of those countries, constantly barraged by mis- and disinformation, you had to keep your guard up. We have a similar propaganda predicament in our society, and we have to be alert and on the lookout. Our desire for quick gratification makes us susceptible to embracing these and other similar myths, lies and disinformation about eating and exercise. Be very aware of self-deception creeping into your mind, and fight it.

BACK TO BASICS

Your best defense against any deception is always go back to the basics of eating and exercise. These basics will never fail you because they are timeless. Back to basics is your best weapon! Then, anytime some "new" eating and exercise tip comes your way, you can immediately test it with your new-found knowledge about the basics of healthy living.

REMEMBER THIS AND AVOID THE MYTHS

- *Eat predominately unprocessed, plant-based foods with approximately 15 % protein, 55 % carbohydrates and 30 % fat.*
- *Limit your intake of animal products to no more than one serving a day -- or, better yet, none at all.*
- *Take a multi-vitamin daily.*
- *Exercise the complete body with cardio, strength and muscle endurance training at least three times per week and, better yet, at least six times per week.*
- *Keep your mind focused on achieving overall health, and you will be effectively able to identify any stealthy attempts by the enemy to distract you with quick fixes.*
- *Focus on overall health and you will achieve a better and more youthful appearance with increased energy.*
- *Focusing on appearance will leave you vulnerable and susceptible to unhealthy and expensive gimmicks and gadgets.*

Chapter Five

Thank God For Hemorrhoids!

A Catalyst For Change

"It's good to have money and the things money can buy, but it's good, too, to check up once in a while and make sure you haven't lost the things money can't buy." - George Horace Lormier

There's a lot of curiosity out there about just what I eat and how I stay in shape. I am going to satisfy that curiosity. The title "Thank God for Hemorrhoids!" has been chosen to catch your attention, but it's not just for the sake of attention-getting. There is a story behind this title which – hopefully – will be an overall health wake-up call for you to make changes and save lives. The life you will be saving will be your own and the lives of others who will observe your healthy lifestyle and become inspired to do the same.

I am not immune to the struggles everyone else has. From time to time, I become a victim of self-deception. All it takes is to allow those enemy soldiers to gain access to your mind and then the excuses open a door that you really don't want open. Don't get me wrong about enjoying those unhealthy, taste-really-good food choices every now and then. That is never the problem. The problem begins when such choices become a part of your routine, your lifestyle, your ongoing habit. The issue is compounded by a sedentary lifestyle, void of exercise.

PASS THE CAKE AND ICE CREAM, PLEASE!

When I was growing up, peanut-butter-and-jelly sandwiches, pancakes with lots of syrup and butter, bacon and sausages were what I fondly remember enjoying. After all, that's what Americans eat, and it must be good for you if they eat it, right? I was certain that these food choices were just plain healthy for me. Thirst-quenchers were juices and Kool-Aid. And when Grandmother would visit, we'd always get an extra helping of ice cream, cookies, cakes and "kisses." I'm sure some of you are familiar with those milk-chocolate bits that are wrapped in a silver, shiny wrapper that are called Kisses. And besides, when I was growing up, being in the country, we were active and always on the move. I played sports, climbed trees, rode a bicycle and walked great distances. No weight problems whatsoever. I was lean and strong. But was I healthy? We also ate fruits and vegetables. We just ate too many sweets, processed foods and animal products.

WHAT DOES IT REALLY TAKE TO EAT HEALTHY?

If you are predominantly eating close-to-nature, plant-based, unprocessed foods, you are probably eating healthy. If, on the other hand, you are predominantly eating processed foods and lots of animal products (meat and dairy), you are probably eating unhealthy.

EAT PLANT-BASED FOODS

Plant-based and unprocessed. Both are key words to remember. My childhood food choices were also plant-based, but they were processed, and therefore very low in nutrients and high in sugar, salt and/or fat. Then, our voracious appetite for meat resulted in essentially consuming meat when we should have been eating nutrient-rich plant products. Meat is low in nutrients, compared to plant products that are unprocessed.

TWENTY POUNDS OVERWEIGHT AND HIGH BLOOD PRESSURE

At the age of 48, I was 20 pounds overweight, weighing in at 185 pounds at 5 ft. 8 ½ inches tall, with high blood pressure and cardio-vascular insufficiency. I was taking prescribed medication for about 10 years up to the age of 48.

Back in high school, I weighed 155 pounds and was active in sports. I wrestled and also participated in track and was a sprinter. After high school, I joined the military and went through basic training, which maintained my weight and fitness level. I was in a unit that did not require a heightened level of fitness. Therefore, I had ample opportunity to put on weight, and the general eating habits were not up to the standards that I have established in this book. My eating habits reflected those of the general U.S. population, and they were not good. I also ended up on the upper limit of what is permissible in the U.S. Army to be within the weight limit. Those standards are not an indicator of good health.

I TOOK INVENTORY OF MY HEALTH AND LIFESTYLE

It was time for my own health assessment. I decided to open my eyes and look around at the people I knew. I looked at how they were living and the health issues they had or didn't have. I found a cause and effect. The health issues of diabetes, high blood pressure, chronic fatigue, heart disease and every cough and cold that passed through the population mostly captured those who led a lifestyle that resulted in these ailments.

Finally, I started to think, "Well, if I start adjusting my eating habits to boost my immune system, this will give me more energy and bring the rest of my body into better balance.

This thought process led to my thinking long-term, five, ten, fifteen and twenty years. I looked at those who were older, with specific ailments, and finally understood that if I continued to live my lifestyle, as it was, without making the changes that I recognized were better for me, I would experience the negative consequences. No wishful thinking will prevent these negative consequences. Only concrete, decisive action will result in improved health and wellbeing.

I GOT SCARED

I scared myself into making some healthy changes. I gradually started backing off of eating fried foods which I had previously enjoyed. A fast-food visit became rare. I consciously sought out fruits, vegetables, whole grains, nuts and beans as the mainstay of my diet. I also began to recognize that these food choices taste fantastic, especially with variety and spices.

Within three months, I lost the extra 20 pounds I had been carrying around for over 20 years. I also discovered, at the age of 48, that I once again was able to sprint like I did in high school. I developed a new-found love for push-ups. My sense of taste and smell perception for healthy food choices improved. The fragrance of a wholesome salad had become superior to my favorite fried dishes with lots of meat.

FOCUS ON APPEARANCE IS A MISTAKE

Since 1999, my mission has been to help others make those healthy lifestyle changes. Along the way, however, I did go through a phase of eating too many chicken breasts and egg whites, which was a deviation from my prime directive to eat predominantly plant-based, and I neglected my diet while emphasizing muscle-building. That was a health mistake. I eventually came back around to health-focused eating predominantly made up of plant-based foods.

And then it happened!

ME WITH HEMORRHOIDS? BUT I EXERCISE!

I got hemorrhoids. I was very fit, but I had slipped back to allowing more processed foods like muffins and bread and pasta and pizza into my diet. My coffee intake had gone from one cup in the morning to two cups in the morning and two cups in the afternoon. It was after a long film shoot on a Sunday. The next morning, I woke up in pain with significant swelling. I was shocked! What? I exercise regularly. This doesn't happen to fit people who exercise, I thought! I went straight to the drugstore to pick up the product I see in those commercials most frequently, Preparation H. I proceeded to walk around the drugstore and could not find it, and I was too embarrassed to ask, so I walked out. Instead, I engaged in some serious research about what had just happened to me.

Here's what I found out about hemorrhoids. Hemorrhoids are swollen veins. Don't worry! I'm leaving out the gory details, so you can read on. There is an important message and lesson that you need to take with you, so keep reading. Hemorrhoids can be caused by sitting or standing for prolonged periods, violent coughing, lifting heavy objects, and many other similar circumstances. Obesity, lack of exercise, liver damage, food allergies and insufficient consumption of fiber-rich foods can also contribute to the formation of hemorrhoids. Over half of all Americans will have had hemorrhoids by the age of fifty.

Nutrition plays a huge role in whether or not we get hemorrhoids. Hemorrhoids are issues with tissue in our bodies. If I contract hemorrhoids due to eating habits, what is happening with the rest of my body? The body is made up of tissue, from skin to internal organs to muscles, tendons and ligaments.

I WENT "COLD TURKEY!"

From one day to the next, I ceased all coffee drinking and any form of processed foods – I was really enjoying those muffins! I went back to basics:

oatmeal with raisins, nuts, fruit and ground flax seeds for breakfast; a salad for lunch with vinegar and olive oil, whole grains and/or potatoes (no animal products!); and a dinner of a starchy carb (rice or potatoes), vegetable and chicken breast (not too much!). I also supplemented with multivitamins, B-complex, calcium, and Vitamins E and C, which were recommended as being very important for tissue building, healing and blood clotting, to target the hemorrhoids.

After four days of this radical change, I went through withdrawal symptoms. I had muscle and joint aches and pains and headaches, none caused by my exercise regimen. I am generally medication-free, but I took a pain-killer to sleep for about two nights. Then it was over. I had no more urge for coffee or for muffins or bread. This stuff really is just like drugs! Don't get me wrong! I may go back to a cup of coffee a day or I may not. I may occasionally eat something like a muffin or I may not. That's the approach and attitude that will not harm your health. Overindulgence and regular indulgence of unhealthy food choices will hurt your health, and could cost you your life or the life of a loved one who sees you doing it and thinks it must be okay.

The hemorrhoids vanished after four weeks. Let me hear an applause! The lifestyle changes kicked the hemorrhoids out of my body.

MARCHING ORDERS – LIFE LESSONS OF A HEMORRHOIDAL ATTACK

Stay away from hemorrhoids! I would like to say I'm joking, but I'm not. Listen carefully to your body. Watch that self-deception mechanism, and constantly work at improving the quality of your life.

After four weeks, the hemorrhoids completely disappeared. And there's more. I am much more alert, and my energy has increased significantly. I was already high energy, but why just go for what is good when you can have the best? When I get up in the morning, my wake-up process is almost immediate. The quality of my sleep has improved. Pain from past injuries also started to dissipate. After six months I've also noticed an improvement in my skin texture, which is an indicator that my internal organs have also started to enjoy the benefit. And now you know the rest of the story.

Thank God for hemorrhoids? You bet! It was just another wake-up call, and I listened and acted upon it. What if it had been a serious form of cancer, or a stroke, or serious heart disease? I am very thankful!

Don't think for one minute that you (or I) become invincible when it comes to slipping back to old ways. When it happens, shout "Cease fire!" Do an about-face, which means turn around for you civilians. Get right back on track. You're worth it.

Remember, everything you do or do not do has consequences, good or bad. It's the long-term consequences that can sneak up on you. Learn to consider the long-term consequences of everything you do and say. Be aware and beware.

Chapter Six

How to Implement a Corporate Wellness Program

Change Your Corporate Culture

80 % of American executives feel that corporate America has a responsibility to promote wellness. - Source: Study by the American Management Association, October 2004

WORKPLACE BEST PLACE FOR WELLNESS PROGRAMS

The work site is one of the best places for health and wellness programs. Employees spend more than half of their waking hours at work. This is an excellent reason to take a close look at how corporate wellness programs can be implemented to increase productivity and revenue while reducing concrete costs related to unhealthy employees.

SMALL BUSINESSES BENEFIT TOO

Small businesses benefit from wellness programs as well. Eliminate any thought from your mind that a wellness program is too expensive. I will show you how to implement a "bare bones," high-impact wellness program that will be affordable for the smallest business.

More and more employers understand that healthy and happy employees are more productive, less stressed, take fewer sick days and care more for and about customers and clients. This chapter will explain how to measure the *return on investment* of wellness programs and how to implement one with very little cost.

There are some employers and employees who may be against workplace wellness programs with the argument, "The workplace is just for work." This would be a fatal view of the workplace since human interaction and productivity at the workplace is made up of much more than just work. There is much more to managing people than just managing work schedules and better performance matrices for improved productivity. Excellent leadership that inspires employees to support one another and care about one another creates a workplace that will benefit from increased productivity and strong, cohesive teams.

IMPLEMENTATION IS PARAMOUNT

Wellness programs in the workplace are not something new. Getting them approved and effectively implemented requires getting past the chief financial officer who is looking for hard facts that will at least result in a break even. If you get $3 back for every $1 invested, you will have achieved an excellent return.

Stronger, healthier and happier Americans are more productive. Inject solid, practiced core and life values into the formula, and the customers and clients will be attracted to your products and services. The corporate wellness program belongs in the arsenal of every business enterprise to increase the bottom line.

THE DILEMMA

Less than 20% of U.S. employers offer lifestyle modification services. 4% offer smoking cessation programs *(2006 study, American Journal of Health Promotion).*

LACK OF WELLNESS PROGRAMS IS COSTING CORPORATIONS BIG BUCKS

The greatest diseases associated with the lack of wellness programs are the following:

> **Sedentary-ītis** – this is the sedentary lifestyle disease.
> **What's-exercise-ītis?** – This is the lack-of-exercise disease.
> **Eat-too-much-ītis** – this one is self-explanatory.
> **Eat-too-much-fat-and-sugar-ītis** – this one is self-explanatory.

These four "diseases" are primary contributors to cost-incurring medical issues. Any program that focuses on overcoming their cost-incurring and time-robbing consequences is the most effective program.

In 2002, a study titled "Economic Costs of Diabetes in the U.S." was conducted. The direct medical and indirect expenditures associated with diabetes for the U.S. population amounted to an estimated $132 billion per year. This costs the U.S. economy an estimated $92 billion on higher health care expenditures. Lost productivity attributed to diabetes resulting from lost workdays, lost home services, permanent disability, and premature death is estimated at $40 billion. Health care spending in 2002 for people with diabetes is more than double what spending would be without diabetes.

Source: Report prepared by Paul Hogan, Tim Dall, and Plamen Nikolov of the Lewin Group, Inc., Falls Church, Virginia; appeared in Diabetes Care, Volume 26, Number 3, March 2003, Report from the American Diabetes Association

Diabetes is the fifth leading cause of death by disease in the United States. Diabetes also contributes to higher rates of occurrence of other diseases. People with diabetes are at higher risk for heart disease, blindness, kidney failure, extremity amputations, and other chronic conditions. See the American Diabetes Association website at Diabetes.org for more information.

According to the Centers for Disease Control, more than 75% of employers' health care costs and productivity losses are related to employee lifestyle choices.

20% ARE RESPONSIBLE FOR 80% OF THE COSTS

AstraZeneca, a pharmaceutical company, determined that 20% of its workforce was responsible for 80% of lost productivity and total health care costs. By focusing on the 20% group, AstraZeneca was able to reduce emergency room visits and hospital admissions.

Source: Forbes.com, "The ROI of Wellness," by Tony Zook, president and chief executive officer of AstraZeneca U.S., April 24, 2006

LIFESTYLE AND HEALTH ISSUES OF WORKING AMERICANS

For every 100 employees nationwide:

60 are sedentary.

25 smoke.

20 are obese.

27 have active cardiovascular disease.

10 have diabetes.

50 have high cholesterol.

24 have high blood pressure.

50 are distressed or depressed.

$510 billion was spent on medical care for chronic conditions in the year2000. By the year 2020, this amount will balloon to over $1 trillion.

Source: The National Center for Health Promotion and Disease Prevention, www.prevention.va.gov

BENEFITS OF A CORPORATE WELLNESS PROGRAM

There are both tangible and intangible benefits to a corporate wellness program. As with any program that is not directly related to revenue producing activities or the primary mission and purpose of the business enterprise, the program is justifiably scrutinized.

Don't be concerned if you are not in a position to track all the data. As long as you are at least tracking those areas and activities that directly impact health and well-being of your employees, you will achieve measurable benefits.

I, too, am dangling the financial benefits carrot with the title "Save Money and Lives with a Corporate Wellness Program" and "The ROI of Corporate Wellness Programs." The truth is that payback and benefits go far beyond simply *Return on Investment.*

TANGIBLE BENEFITS

Reductions in sick leave absenteeism

Reduced use of health benefit

Reduced workers' compensation

Reduced injury experience

Reduced presenteeism losses

INTANGIBLE BENEFITS

Improvements in employee morale
Increased employee loyalty
Less organizational conflict
More productive work force
Improved employee decision-making ability
Improved employee retention

CORE WELLNESS COMPONENTS

A wellness program that includes the physical, social, occupational, intellectual, spiritual and emotional components is a program that addresses the true needs of employees. Address employee needs and you will enhance health and performance. My Corporate Fitness Boot Camp Program is designed to address all six of the following wellness components. See the chapter titled "How to Organize Your Own Fitness Boot Camp" for more details.

Physical – body, endurance, flexibility, strength
Social – family, friends, relationships
Occupational – personal and professional development, worthwhile work
Intellectual – mind, creativity, knowledge
Spiritual – values, purpose, religion, intuition
Emotional – feelings, self-esteem, coping with stress

Source: Veterans Health Administration (VHA) Employee Wellness Program Start-Up Guide, page 4, National Center for Health Promotion and Disease Prevention and The Wellness Advisory Council

WHAT TO MEASURE TO DETERMINE THE ROI OF WELLNESS PROGRAMS

Worker's compensation claims – number and dollar value
Absenteeism – Sick days used, while factoring out exceptions such as family leave.
Presenteeism – This refers to the cost of employees who are at work but not functioning at their full capacity. There are three basic types of questions that can be asked:
- o "On average, how many days each month are you limited at work due to back pain, headaches, head colds, or other illnesses?"

    o   "On average, how many days each month are you limited at work due to family issues, financial concerns, or other work/life balance issues?"

    o   "On those days, at what percent of your normal ability are you able to function? – 10% - 30% - 50% - 70% - 90%."

Number of injuries and light duty time

Health insurance expenditures

Health indicators – such as weight/BMI, cardio, strength, blood pressure, lipids, fasting blood sugar levels, tobacco usage, reported health behaviors, diagnosis or family histories of heart disease, hypertension, diabetes, and cancers. These can be obtained voluntarily through screenings and the use of Health Risk Appraisals.

Source: VHA Employee Wellness Program Start-Up Guide, National Center for Health Promotion and Disease Prevention and The Wellness Advisory Council

INCENTIVES AND POSITIVE ENCOURAGEMENT

There are many incentives that can be used to get employees to actively improve their health and wellness. The primary purpose of incentives should be to increase participation.

Some incentives to participate in wellness events and programs could be:

Cash
Refreshments
Give-aways
Discounts
Drawings
Recognition
Time off
Education/training time

POSITIVE CORPORATE CULTURE IS KEY TO A LASTING AND SUCCESSFUL WELLNESS PROGRAM

A values-based corporate culture that demonstrates a sense of caring for the employees as well as the customers and clients is fundamental for a successful corporate wellness program. Any wellness program instituted needs to convey to the employees that their employer cares about their health and well-being. A wellness program that conveys a sense of being predominantly a means of increasing revenue and productivity is not a program that will last. A part of this corporate culture is the employees caring about the health and well-being of each other. That ensures an excellent support system, which also enhances team spirit. An employee who feels that his employer and fellow employees care about his well-being is a happy and more productive employee and is more apt to support and help other employees.

IMPLEMENTATION IS IMPERATIVE

How easy is it to implement a wellness program? I'll show you. Get down in the push-up position right now. Knock out five push-ups. If you can only perform partial push-ups, you have still implemented fitness. You can actually implement a program quickly and affordably. My chapter on "How to Organize Your Own Fitness Boot Camp" will tell you how. This is not an oversimplification. It is that easy to implement a wellness program with maximum impact on the health and well-being of your employees. Just do it!

Whether an employer has a small or large business enterprise, implementation of a wellness program is imperative. A no-excuses approach must be taken to save employees from suffering and death, all the while enjoying the benefit of increased productivity. It makes no difference how well you are able to track and monitor the *Return on Investment*. Do not let the implementation of an employee wellness program fall by the wayside simply because you are lacking resources to track the data. Do not let your plan for an employee wellness program become another file gathering dust. The wellness program is too critical to ignore. If you do nothing else except focus on physical fitness and healthy eating, you will have a very significant impact on the health and well-being of your employees and your company.

BUY-IN IS ESSENTIAL

It makes no difference whether the initiative for a workplace wellness program comes from senior or mid-level management or from line employees. Buy-in is needed from all levels of your business.

HOW TO GET BUY-IN FROM EMPLOYEES AND MANAGEMENT

Internal sales and marketing skills are the key to creating buzz and excitement about a workplace wellness program. At the end of this chapter, you will find more resources to make it easy to present convincing arguments to fit your business enterprise, whether you are a small business or a large corporation.

A "bare bones" implemented wellness program includes the following:

Exercise
Healthy eating
Health and fitness screening

The high-impact wellness program that has immediate and long-term benefits is the implementation of a fitness program and/or programs. Two fitness programs that you, as the employer, can implement this week are "Organize Your Own Fitness Boot Camp" and the "M.O.V.E.™ Kick-start Exercise and Weight-loss Program." Both programs are covered in this book.

WELLNESS PROGRAM RESOURCES

EXERCISE

TheHealthColonel.com
HealthierUS.gov. The source of credible, accurate information to help Americans choose to live healthier lives.
NutritionData.com. The quickest way to find out what's good and bad about the foods you eat.
Presidentschallenge.org
Fitness.org, The President's Council on Physical Fitness and Sports

HEALTHY EATING

See the chapter on "Six Keys to Permanent Weight-loss" for basic guidelines on eating healthy. There are lots of resources that can be used. Some of them are:

Your health insurance company
Wellness-related non-profit organizations
Local hospitals
Local nutritionists
Weight Watchers representative
Health Finder at Healthfinder.gov
Handouts at Move.va.gov/Handouts.asp

American Diabetes Association, Diabetes.org

HEALTH SCREENING AND ASSESSMENT

Lifeline Screening: www.lifelinescreening.com
MedLinePlus: www.nlm.nih.gov/medlineplus/healthscreening.html
www.ahrq.gov/ppip/adguide/checkups.htm
Adult Preventive Care Timeline: www.ahrq.gov/ppip/timelinead.pdf
Your health insurance company
Red Cross
Local hospitals
Health assessment survey questionnaire:
www.prevention.va.gov/Wellness/HealthAssessmentSurvey_2006.doc
General health and disease assessment:
www.houston.med.va.gov/PatientEd/HealthInfo/General_Health_and_Dis
ease_Risk_Assessment.asp
American Diabetes Association: Diabetes.org

OTHER WELLNESS ASSOCIATIONS

National Association for Health and Fitness. The National Association
for Health and Fitness (NAHF) is a non-profit organization that exists to
improve the quality of life for individuals in the United States through the
promotion of physical fitness, sports and healthy lifestyles.
The National Wellness Association.
www.nationalwellnessassociation.com
The American Association of Occupational Health Nurses.
www.aaohn.org The mechanism for success or failure is no different from
any other goals (weight-loss, eat right, further education, go to church,
save money, improve marriage, more personal and professional
development).

The implemented wellness program is not just for those periodic meetings
reserved for a little discussion with a wink and nod (= "Not a priority. Next?) from
management.

MANY BUSINESSES HAVE ACHIEVED GREAT RESULTS

There are lots of excellent examples of a significant return on investment and improved health of employees as well as increased productivity. In a study funded by the Centers for Disease Control (CDC), a federal agency, and conducted by Dr. Ron Goetzl, Cornell University, it was determined that a 1% improvement through a wellness program can result in a $3 ROI for every $1 invested.

EXAMPLES OF RETURNS OF WELLNESS PROGRAM INVESTMENTS

- **Dow Chemical** achieved a 0.17% improvement to break even. A 1% improvement resulted in a $50 million savings.
- **Motorola** achieved 0.67% improvement to break even.
- **Union Pacific** achieved a 0.49% improvement to break even.
- **PepsiCo** achieved $3 for every $1 invested.
- **General Mills** achieved $3.90 for every $1 invested.
- **Citibank** achieved $4.56 to $4.73 for every $1 invested.

WELLNESS TOOL KIT

The Department of Veterans Affairs - The National Center for Health Promotion and Disease Prevention - has an excellent tool kit to help start a wellness program at www.prevention.va.gov/Wellness_Toolkit.asp.

MARCHING ORDERS – SAVE MONEY AND LIVES WITH A CORPORATE WELLNESS PROGRAM – CHANGE YOUR EMPLOYEES' HEALTH

- *Plan and present the benefits of your corporate wellness program.*
- *Implement the basics of physical exercise and healthy eating within four weeks of planning.*
- *All leaders of your company will implement their own personal wellness programs and publish them so that all employees understand that their leaders take health and wellness seriously.*
- *Organize your own fitness boot camp cells/teams and implement within four weeks.*
- *Conduct first fitness test within four weeks and establish fou- week goals based on the chapter, "Fitness Goals and Progress Measurement – Change with Goals."*
- *Use local resources to support a measurable, healthy eating and exercise program.*
- *Make exercise and healthy eating a part of personal and professional development.*

- *Praise effort and reward performance.*
- *Create incentives and awards.*
- *Celebrate as a team the gains and goal accomplishments.*
- *Set the standard and let every employee know that your company is a company of healthy lifestyles.*
- *Integrate as many core wellness components into your programs as possible.*
- *Understand that whether or not a wellness program to save lives and suffering of those under your supervision is implemented cannot be optional. There is a moral and leadership responsibility.*
- *As Winston Churchill said, "Men occasionally stumble over the truth, but most pick themselves up and hurry off as if nothing happened." Don't let this happen to you.*

Nothing great has ever been achieved except by those who dared believe something inside them was superior to circumstances.

- Bruce Barton

Chapter Seven

How to Organize Your Own Fitness Boot Camp

Change How You Workout

Make fitness boot camp a part of your corporate culture and you will build strong teams, increase productivity and change the lives of your employees. - Lt. Col. Bob Weinstein, USAR (ret.)

It's time to successfully organize and conduct your own fitness boot camp program. Pay careful attention. This chapter is not some nice-to-read theoretical information that never gets implemented. Read this with one thing in mind: a firm decision to implement this program. My intent is to save lives and prevent suffering from disease and illness. Make this your intent.

WHO IS THE HEALTH COLONEL'S FITNESS BOOT CAMP FOR?

Fitness boot camp is designed for all ages, all sizes and shapes, as well as all fitness levels. It is great for beginners and those who have never exercised before as well as for the regular exerciser. Although the focus of this chapter is on the business environment, the same approach can be applied to families, friends, schools, clubs and associations looking for a fun way to work out together.Fitness boot camp will enhance existing wellness and fitness programs. I also offer a video series that will allow you to see me in action with the "troops," so that you get a better visual of what I am talking about.

PERFECT FOR BUSY SCHEDULES

You will learn how – with little or no cost – to organize your very own fitness boot camp cells/teams. I call this the busy person's workout, because it covers the strength, cardio and flexibility all wrapped into one workout session. As always, consult with your physician before beginning this or any other fitness activity. See the chapter on the M.O.V.E.™ Fitness and Weight-loss Program to add a

heightened   level of accountability for all new participants, employees and/or recruits for the first four months.

WHAT YOU GET WITH THE HEALTH COLONEL'S FITNESS BOOT CAMP

Variety.

Fun.

Energizing.

Builds strong teams.

Incorporates company, family and life core values.

Complete-body, encompassing strength, muscle endurance, flexibility and cardio.

Can be started anytime.

No strict work-out regimen.

Dynamic, always focused on progress.

Can be done indoors and/or outdoors.

For men, women, teens and children.

For pre-beginners, beginners, intermediates and advanced.

For young and old.

This workout is for the company looking for a creative way of getting its employees in shape while strengthening team spirit, increasing productivity and reducing absenteeism.

The purpose of implementing the Health Colonel's™ Fitness Boot Camp Cells/Teams is to actively take on the role of getting employees, club members, family members and friends in shape and build strong, cohesive teams.

WORKPLACE BENEFITS OF THE HEALTH COLONEL'S FITNESS BOOT CAMP

Little to no cost.

Use existing employee and management structure to organize.

Enhancement of corporate culture.

Healthier and happier employees.

Enhanced team spirit.

Reduced illnesses.

Reduced loss of work time.

Reduced injuries.

Increased productivity and performance.

Weight-loss and weight management.

Nutritional guidance.

Stress relief and stress management.

Enhanced communication.

APPOINT TEAM LEADERS

Appoint team leaders for each cell, which will be made up of approximately six to twenty employees. This is a company-wide approach, from senior management all the way down to front-line employees. Any member of management can simply step in and join the workout with any of the teams to further promote their relationships with employees while working on their own fitness and demonstrating, by example, how important this is. Management participation is a non-threatening way for senior- and mid-level management to join in on what is offered as "serious fun" with special emphasis on fun and teambuilding.

Decide on how best to organize your initial team cells and appoint teamleaders or coordinators (one for each cell). Then, assign one individual to support all team coordinators of all the cells and to track the programs. That individual could be the wellness coordinator, supervisor, manager or some other employee. That individual should already possess a heightened level of enthusiasm for fitness and have a desire to help others.

DIFFERENT FITNESS LEVELS TRAIN TOGETHER

All fitness levels train together. Have all employees sign a waiver for the program. If any members have medical issues, those employees would then only perform those exercises that are permissible by their physician; for example, walking but no jogging, no ab work, no squats or lunges due to knee injury. Often a simple modification of an exercise is possible. Those with medical restrictions would then perform their alternative exercises during the time the rest of the team is performing their (unmodified) exercise; or they will simply modify the team's exercise to a safe range of motion suitable to their medical limitation.

ORGANIZE FITNESS CELLS

Those employees who work together on a regular basis should be organized as a part of the same fitness cell. You can organize the cells by department or cross-departmental. Have managers or peers come together; mix various management levels. Rearrange the mix of employees every six months, if you desire. Whether your business is customer service, sales, banking, law office staff, fire and rescue, hospital staff, law enforcement, school, college or university, or small business with a handful of employees, boot camp fitness cells are right for you.

INDOORS OR OUTDOORS

Another exciting aspect of fitness boot camp is these workouts can be done anywhere, whether indoors or outdoors. Keep it interesting by changing workout location, where feasible, and look for opportunities to incorporate your environment into your workout. For example, park benches are great for performing dips, and the entire team can wrap their resistance Bands around a tree for a group upper-body exercise.

FLEXIBLE

You choose a time to fit your schedule. Whether it's 10, 20, 30 or 60 minutes for fitness boot camp, it all adds up to an accumulative health benefit. I strongly recommend at least twice a week, once a week at a minimum, as a part of a corporate program with emphasis that the employees work out four to six times per week all told. If you can't schedule fitness boot camp twice a week, schedule the frequency that will work. Make it a part of your corporate culture, and your employees will take this into their private fitness routines. There is a clear connection between fitness and workplace performance.

COMBINE WORKOUT WITH A BUSINESS MEETING

Combine a meeting with fitness boot camp. There is no better way to get those creative juices flowing while problem solving than to engage in hearty exercise. Start off with an issue to be considered or a problem to be solved, and then perform an exercise or two. Stop and discuss. Then do it again with the next agenda point, until all issues and muscle groups have been addressed. Who says you can't combine work with pleasure? Yeah, that's right! I said pleasure!

ANYONE CAN DO IT

The training is easy, and the exercises are very basic and easy to perform. The mix of exercises follows the principles of simplicity and fun. Technically, this is called functional training. Functional training focuses on training the body how it is used in activities of daily life.

TRAIN THE TRAINERS

Once you've identified your trainers, they need to be trained. To immediately implement this program the trainers will only need a few basic exercises. Start off with these basics and, with time, gradually introduce new exercises. The trainers are not just watching. They are performing the exercises with their team members as they guide and encourage them through the workout.

THREE BASIC PRINCIPLES

1. **Warm-up.** Perform toe raisers to warm up the body.
2. **Stretch.** Stretch each body part briefly right after exercising it.
3. **Strength and cardio.** Alternate between upper and lower body exercises.

This approach is safe and does not require much training to implement. Participants are to stay in touch with their bodies and do only what they can do. If they can only perform a partial motion of an exercise, that is acceptable and is still working the muscles. Use the following list of basic exercises to get started. You will find a description of these exercises in Part Two of this book.

START WITH THESE EXERCISES

Squats
Standing crunches

Standing lunge
Arms and shoulders stretch
Triceps and upper back stretch
Standing straddle and stretch
Standing hamstring stretch
Biceps curls, resistance band
Shoulder press, resistance band
Upright row, resistance band
Crunches

GROUND RULES FOR FITNESS BOOT CAMP

There are ground rules to follow. These rules are designed to build strong, supportive teams and team members. Focus on the basic approach of the workout, to guarantee progress for all team members, all while having lots of fun.

SAFETY

Keep the workouts safe. Ask about medical restrictions and remind participants to stay in touch with their own bodies. The workout is designed to take the employees out of their comfort zone periodically so that fitness progress can be experienced. The comfort zone will differ for each individual. A team member only modifies an exercise for medical reasons or due to fatigue level and then continues to exercise that body part.

DO NOT allow the question of liability to cause the program to be rejected or terminated. The advantages of this fitness program far outweigh any questions of risk or liability. Seek legal counsel to mitigate any risk. Require all participants to stay in touch with their own bodies and do only what they can do.

SIMPLICITY

I've already talked about the principle of simplicity. As a team progresses, new exercises can be incorporated into the workout, periodically changing the routine, location or sequence of exercises. Introducing something new keeps it interesting.

FUN

The fun factor cannot be emphasized enough. The workouts are all performed in a light, upbeat and positive atmosphere with an emphasis on mutual respect and concern for all team members. Humor is an important element, as long as it is not demeaning or inappropriate in language or content. No foul language is to be used by any team member. Treat the workout like a game and have a blast!

VARIETY

Variety is the spice of life. And variety is one of the principles that keeps the workout interesting and actually plays a role in "surprising" the neurological system into supporting greater fitness progress.

COMPLETE BODY WORKOUT

Complete body workout means strength, cardio and flexibility. It also means upper body, lower body and abs. Every workout will include all of these in varying degrees. This is easy to apply. Simply spoken, what you will do is: jog or walk; stop and work a body part; jog or walk; stop and work a body part -- until the entire session is complete.

Are you indoors and can't go outdoors? Be creative and perform the exercises while alternating between upper and lower body. I can assure you, you will get a cardio workout as well. Every session may have a different emphasis. For example, the upper body may be emphasized, while the other areas are still being worked. The order of exercises may be random, as long as there is a switching off between upper and lower body.

CORE VALUES

The core values of the company are to be consciously practiced and illustrated during the workouts. Core values are designed to make us better employees and better persons. For example, the core values of the U.S. Army are loyalty, duty, respect, selfless-service, honor, integrity and personal courage. A clear understanding of the company core values is an essential part of the training. During each training session, a particular core value or values should be emphasized to talk about. This can be accomplished by selecting an appropriate quote or quotes or a life or business scenario or anecdote that best demonstrates the core value.

ENHANCE WORKPLACE PERFORMANCE

The practice of core values of a company is very important for the long-term success of the company and for great employer/employee and employee/customer relations.

All people have different skill sets and different levels of performance. The object of fitness boot camp is to make all team members feel appreciated and motivated regardless of performance levels. That is a huge secret to enhancing the performance of all.

Team members will all have different fitness levels. Some will have stronger upper bodies, some will have greater flexibility, and some will have better cardio. Each team member focuses on his or her individual fitness progress based on his or her very own fitness level and not the fitness level of other team members. All team members support each other in their individual quests to improve. Fitness boot camp is not only about physical strength, it is also about mental strength.

MENTAL FORTITUDE

Mental fortitude pushes us to improve and go beyond our present fitness level. In order to improve the mental fortitude, 100 % effort is required of all team members. 100 % effort means that if a team member, during the course of an exercise, gets so fatigued that the complete exercise cannot be performed, then that team member will not simply quit, but will modify the exercise to the point of being able to continue. Without a struggle, there can be no progress! This is where the mental fortitude is actually being strengthened again along with the body. Strengthening of mental fortitude will carry over into the workplace. This is very powerful. This keeps the mind and body in the mode of saying, "Hey, I can do this! I won't stop! I won't quit!" This is what adds the challenge to the fun.

COUNT REPS OUT LOUD TOGETHER

All team members will count exercises with repetitions out loud and enthusiastically. No exceptions except for laryngitis and those who cannot speak. This works the diaphragm and also has a very positive team-building impact on team members. If you want to experience how I conduct a class, you can order one of my workout videos, available at my website, NoMoreCryBabies.com. If you happen to be in an environment that will disturb others by counting out loud, whisper instead.

MARCHING ORDERS – HOW TO ORGANIZE YOUR OWN FITNESS BOOT CAMP

- *Implement this program and don't let "busy-ness" get in the way. The stakes are too high and the benefits too great.*
- *Make this program a part of your corporate culture.*
- *Create ranks with incentives to get promoted to the next rank.*
- *Celebrate all progress of team members.*
- *Create awards to recognize special achievers in the area of weight-loss and fitness and nutrition.*
- *Report to the Health Colonel the formation of your fitness team at TheHealthColonel@BeachBootCamp.net.*
- *Establish and measure short-term and long-term fitness, nutrition and team-building goals.*
- *Sign up for my free newsletter at www.TheHealthColonel.com.*

Contact me with any questions you may have about organizing your fitness boot camp at 888.768.9892 or email me at: TheHealthColonel@BeachBootCamp.net.

You are not beaten until you admit it.

- George S. Patton

Chapter Eight

Weight-loss Program M.O.V.E.™

Kick-start Change

"An object at rest tends to stay at rest and an object in motion tends to stay in motion." - Sir Isaac Newton

We all need a little push or kick-start to get things going. The four month M.O.V.E.™ fitness and weight-loss program is designed to create momentum in achieving your worthy goals of weight-loss and/or improving on your fitness and health. Isaac Newton's First Law of Physics applies here. You are the object he's talking about being in motion or at rest, whichever the case may be. If you are mostly leading a sedentary lifestyle – well, you are that object at rest that tends to stay at rest, which explains why it is so difficult to get some motion going. If you are that object in motion, your tendency is predetermined by the law of physics; your tendency is to remain in motion. My objective is to get that object (you) at rest to move, so that that object (you) stays in motion and on the M.O.V.E.™

THE WEIGHT-LOSS/MANAGEMENT PROGRAM M.O.V.E. ™ STANDS FOR

M aximize your results.
O vercome your weaknesses and bad habits.
V ictory is assured through lifestyle change empowerment.
E nergize your body.

The Problem: Extra Pounds, Sedentary Lifestyle, Bad Eating Habits

Are you looking to fit into that special dress? (I'm talkin' about the ladies here -- or need I mention that?)
Are you looking to reverse the signs of aging?
Are you having problems getting rid of that excess weight?
Do you just want to look great in that new bikini?
Are you ready to get that toned and firm body you have always wanted?
Are you out of shape and getting more so?
Don't know how to break those bad eating habits?
Don't have time to exercise?
Are you seeking to simply improve your fitness level?
Are you looking to improve your health?

The Solution: Your Own Fitness And Weight-Loss M.O.V.E.™ Program

You can organize the M.O.V.E. program as an integral part of your fitness boot camp team or cell or at your gym, or you can just pair up using a buddy system. Some of the assessments may be beyond your expertise or beyond the expertise of your team members. That's okay. Check with your local gym, club or wellness coordinator.

You may also e-mail me with any questions or feedback at TheHealthColonel@BeachBootCamp.net.

THE M.O.V.E.™ PROGRAM INCLUDES:

Weight-Loss Goals Established – You should not lose more than one to two pounds per week.

Eating Habits Assessed – Perform a self-assessment or have a team member help you and apply the basics as set forth in this book on eating for performance and energy.

Eating Issues Identified – The basic issues are either quantity and/or quality of food.

Eating and Fitness Action Plan – Create a plan of exercise three to six days per week and put it in your calendar like a doctor's appointment you must attend or like a project assigned by your boss that you must complete.

Body Mass Index (BMI) – Go to Diabetes.org of the American Diabetes Association to calculate your BMI online every four weeks. You'll find excellent tips for eating and exercise plans at Diabetes.org whether you have diabetes or not.

- **Body Measurements** taken every four weeks – Use a tailor's tape measure to take body measurements.
- **Fitness Test** every four weeks (Total of five fitness tests including initial testing). The test: Push-ups, crunches (or sit-ups) and a one-mile run and/or walk. For fitness testing see the chapter titled "Fitness Goals and Progress Measurement."
- **Fitness Goals** established every four weeks – Based on your fitness tests.
- **Digital Photos** taken for before-and-after photos – Smile as you get into shape!
- **Email support:** You may e-mail me at TheHealthColonel@BeachBootCamp.net with any questions you may have or call me toll-free at 888.768.9892.

M.O.V.E. is the catalyst you need to make those lifestyle changes that will encompass all those areas of your life that are truly important to you. Feel and visualize the new you with the following benefits:

- Healthy weight and size.
- Sleep better at night.
- More brain power due to reduced stress.
- More energy to keep going.
- Master life planning skills to keep on track with what is best for your happiness.
- Heightened level of awareness about how to lead a healthy life.

MARCHING ORDERS – M.O.V.E.™ WEIGHT-LOSS PROGRAM

- *Find a buddy or trainer to administer the fitness tests and take the measurements.*
- *Establish your four-week goals once the fitness test is administered.*
- *The fitness test events are push-ups, crunches or sit-ups, and a one-mile run/walk. See chapter titled "Fitness Goals and Progress Measurement" for details.*
- *Record all measurements to include your height, weight and age. See chapter titled "Fitness Goals and Progress Measurement" for details.*

- *Do this for at least four months, and you will experience improvement in your fitness. To experience the necessary weight-loss, adjust the quantity and quality of food you are eating.*

If you should have questions contact Colonel Bob at: TheHealthColonel@BeachBootCamp.net or at his website at: TheHealthColonel.com or call toll-free at: 888.768.9892

Chapter Nine

Who is Responsible for the Health Crisis in America?

Change the Health Crisis

A baby born in the U.S. in 2004 will live an average of 77.9 years. That life expectancy ranks 42d in the world, down from 11th twenty years earlier. - Source: Census Bureau and National Center for Health Statistics

BLAME-STORMING THE HEALTH CRISIS

Who is responsible for the health crisis in America? Is it the government? The state of the economy? Parents? Schools? What about you and me? Restaurants? Grocery stores? Or is it our busy schedules? How about those get-togethers and parties you attend? Maybe the presented food choices are to blame. Yes! "Blame." That's the word I was looking for! We're looking for someone or some institution to blame for our health crisis.

IS THERE A GOVERNMENT CONSPIRACY?

Or is there a government conspiracy? If so, just who are the conspirators? Let's get one thing straight. You and I do not need anyone's help in creating a health crisis. There's a reason for this. You and I are the greatest conspirators of our own lives. We have received more than enough information to let us know what to do to enhance our health and yet we, in many cases, don't act and make the changes. I think that clarifies the conspiracy theory in a nutshell. So anytime you want to blame someone else or some institution, cease fire! Cease that thought!

When I speak of this health crisis, I am not talking about medical insurance or medical costs or treatment. True, this is an important issue. But this issue only touches on the surface of the problem. How we think, eat and live is the real cause. So who or what is responsible? Do you have an idea? Who is the villain or culprit?

YOU ARE RESPONSIBLE FOR YOUR HEALTH

You are personally responsible for all the decisions you make. That stands firm. Do not blame any institution or anyone else for your poor choices that lead to disease, illness and poor health.

WHY AMERICANS RANK LOW ON LONGEVITY

What has caused America to fall so far behind the statistics on longevity in the world? The ranking went from 11th to 42d. Americans do live longer, but not as long as 41 other countries, according to National Center on Health Statistics. Why is one of the richest countries in the world not able to keep up with other countries?

Some say it is because the United States has no universal health care. I don't see that as the *primary* reason since we have never had universal health care.

Here's what I think are some of the primary reasons for this trend:

> Adults in the United States have one of the highest obesity rates in the world. One third of U.S. adults 20 years and older are obese and about two thirds are overweight, according to the National Center for Health Statistics.
> Americans are extremely sedentary in their lifestyles.
> Americans don't exercise at all or very little.
> Americans eat too much and they eat too much processed foods, sugar and fat.
> As long as the health care debate is limited to insurance, the health of Americans will not improve.

SAM MADE ME DO IT

Kids sometimes will do the craziest things. Once upon a time, there were two brothers. We'll call them Sam and Jake. As school-aged brothers, Sam challenged Jake to climb a tree, and so he does. Then Jake is challenged, on a dare, to go farther out on a long, thin branch of the tree. He gets about half way out before the limb breaks, and he comes falling to the earth with a thump. Jake broke his nose and got some cuts and bruises. Both kids report to their mother and of course Mom asks Jake, "How did this happen?" Jake responds, "Sam made me do it!"

There are lots of complaints I hear about all that enticing processed food in the grocery stores. There are remarks about the special challenge of eating out: The portion sizes are too big, and there are all those irresistible, unhealthy "choices" available. I see no difference between Jake's response and these complaining adults' reactions to their plight – or, should I say, dilemma. Jake said, "Sam made me do it." Translation: Sam is responsible for Jake's poor decision to go out on a limb. That's nonsense. Jake is responsible for his own decision to go out on a limb. We adults are too frequently "going out on a limb" with our health by making poor choices while laying the blame on external circumstances or institutions -- whether commercial, social, or governmental. Cease fire with such thoughts of blaming external circumstances or other people. Take charge. Be accountable for your own actions.

INSTITUTIONAL RESPONSIBILITY

Are our institutions off the hook when it becomes to responsibility? No, they are not. I use the term "institution" in a broad sense, to include the following:

Federal, state and local governments
Political parties and politicians
Teachers and school boards
Physicians, dentists, nurses
Journalists, press and media
CEO's and corporate shareholders
Restaurateurs, marketers
School cafeterias
Workplace cafeterias
Clergy, little league coaches
Parents and caregivers
Law enforcement officers, parole officers
Military leaders (from the squad leader upward)

WHAT DO THESE AND OTHER INSTITUTIONS ALL HAVE IN COMMON?

Tradition
Cultural power
Authority over others' behavior
Influence

INSTITUTIONS ARE RESPONSIBLE TO LEAD BY EXAMPLE

What kind of leadership responsibility do institutions have when it comes to healthy eating and exercise? Institutions, as well as all leaders, have a heightened level of responsibility beyond rules and regulations of the organization.

Our institutions have the special responsibility to "walk the talk," clarify the goals of health and fitness, and assume a more visionary role to set and implement standards for a solution to our health crisis. Our institutions are morally obligated to set the example by living by the higher standard required of them as leaders.

This can be accomplished through legislation, executive orders and both internal and public policy making. Our institutions need to take the bull by the horns and use their special influence to save lives and prevent suffering.

HEALTH INSURANCE DOES NOT EQUATE TO A HEALTHY LIFESTYLE OR GOOD HEALTH

Health insurance will not accomplish this. Are you looking for true medical insurance? Make your premium payments in the form of living a healthy lifestyle void of dependence on a home pharmacy of medications. Most of our medications are prescribed because of our lifestyles, not because we simply got sick. I am talking about the overwhelming rule and not the exception.

There are exceptional cases where, despite a healthy lifestyle, serious disease or illness happens. Would you cease to drive a car simply because someone had an automobile accident? Of course not! And you certainly should not cease to lead a healthy lifestyle just because someone you know lived to be 100 years old as a smoker. That would be a fatal error in thinking. It is just this type of thinking that is killing and maiming Americans. Cease fire! Ban this type of thinking from your mind.

Take the educational institutions for America's young people. Schools are primarily focused on delivering on educating our youth with an approved curriculum. Schools need to go beyond mere curriculum, to consider the whole child, setting improved fitness and healthy eating as a priority. Fitness and healthy eating should be a part of the curriculum, as they play a major role in the development of a child.

TEACHERS ARE ROLE MODELS

Teachers are role models and leaders when it comes to eating and exercise habits and how they portray their attitudes about fitness and health in school. In the New York Times Best Seller, "21 Irrefutable Laws of Leadership", John Maxwell defines leadership as "influence - nothing more, nothing less." Moving beyond the position of the teacher to assessing the ability of the teacher to influence others as a leader is essential. This refers to those who would consider themselves followers, and those outside that circle.

Leadership builds character, because without maintaining integrity and trustworthiness, the capability to positively influence will disappear. There are many other definitions of leadership. They all point to a leader having influence on others and providing to them the guidance and direction necessary to envision a long-term view of the future.

POINT OUR CHILDREN IN THE RIGHT DIRECTION

Policy is made from the top down through legislation, executive order, mission and policy statements. Where there is a void in such top-down leadership, the initiative must begin from the ground up.

Educational institutions by virtue of their access to vast blocks of our children's time, have a unique responsibility to go beyond mere curriculum to consider the whole child. By offering and stressing healthier choices, they are setting precedent for the rest of that child's life.

Early in America's pioneer history, schoolteachers were expected to be morally beyond reproach in every detail of their own lifestyle. This reflected how those communities wanted to influence their children's future and the future of the country as a whole. Today's America likewise needs today's schoolteachers to be wholeheartedly health conscious for the same reason. Our future depends on it.

That is not to say that all schoolteachers should be fashion-model thin or good-looking or in any way shaped by the media's image. An overweight teacher who is working to improve her fitness would be preferable over the Size Four who is proud to eat candy bars and drink sodas in front of her pupils.

"Institutions are role models in all that they say and do or do not say or do. Their policies and actions set the standards." - *Lt. Col. Bob Weinstein, USAR (ret.)*

WE ARE KILLING OUR CHILDREN

Take a look at some statistics on childhood obesity in America.

About 15 percent of children and adolescents ages 6-19 years are seriously overweight.

The percentage of children and adolescents who are defined as overweight has nearly tripled since the early 1970s.

Over 10 percent of preschool children between ages two and five are overweight.

Another 15 percent of children and teens ages 6-19 are considered at risk of becoming overweight.

Researchers found that lowered self-esteem was associated with being overweight in girls as young as five.

One in five children in the U.S. is overweight.

Children ages 10-13 who are obese are expected to have a 70% likelihood of suffering from obesity as adults.

Centers for Disease Control and Prevention's (CDC), 1999-2000 National Health and Nutrition Examination Survey (NHANES)

CHILDHOOD OBESITY ONLY AN INDICATOR AND NOT THE REAL PROBLEM

Childhood obesity is only the indicator of an underlying problem of a sedentary lifestyle and unhealthy eating habits. Address these underlying issues, and childhood obesity will also be significantly reduced.

SCHOOLS, TEACHERS AND PARENTS HAVE A HEIGHTENED LEVEL OF RESPONSIBILITY

Our schools, teachers and parents have a heightened level of leadership responsibility to address these statistics that are just a few of many indicators of the direction of the state of health of our children. Once these children become adults, they, too, will pass on their lifestyles to their children and will in all likelihood perpetuate poor eating and exercise habits. The consequences will manifest themselves as learning disabilities, increased crime, and socioeconomic problems which our children's generation cannot afford to inherit.

THE MOTHER OF ALL INSTITUTIONAL EXCUSES

What is the number one excuse institutions use for not doing more to fight the poor state of health of Americans?

Answer: It's each individual's own decision as to how he or she wants to live, how he or she wants to eat and exercise or not.

Cease fire! Wrong answer! This is the Mother of all institutional excuses. An institution using this excuse relinquishes its leadership responsibility as a visionary to lead and guide by example and exercise that institutional influence it possesses. The institutions need to ask the visionary question of what can they do to influence, guide and inspire each individual to make healthy lifestyle choices.

WHY PYRAMIDS AND DIETARY GUIDELINES DON'T WORK

Dietary guidelines, pyramids and charts have all failed to make Americans healthier. Why are they not working? Institutions are made up of individuals who are a cross-section of society who are therefore personally dealing with the same lifestyle issues about eating and exercise as are all consumers.

Dietary guidelines do not work, because the vast majority of the food and beverage industry does not incorporate them into food choices and portion sizes we see on the shelves. Remember, this is from the perspective of the institution and its responsibility and in no way diminishes the personal responsibility of every individual to take charge of their own lifestyle and choices. Our children need special guidance to learn what personal responsibility means. That guidance must come from adults.

GOVERNMENT SETS THE STANDARD AS A LEADER

Emission controls in the automobile industry have resulted in smaller, cleaner, and more fuel-efficient cars; though more work remains to be done. These successes were accomplished through government regulation through the Clean Air Act and similar initiatives. We have another just as pressing form of pollution going on in America: health pollution.

HEALTH POLLUTION

We have a health pollution crisis on our hands in America, and – as with automobile emission regulations – the food and beverage industry needs to be regulated to meet improved standards for healthy eating through strict labeling, reduced portion sizes, and regulation and disclosure of unhealthy ingredients in our country's food supply.

The free market society needs some governmental fine tuning in order to save American lives and prevent suffering. The cost of not doing so is enormous. Heart disease, cancer, stroke, and diabetes (the four leading causes of death in the U.S.), and also obesity, hypertension, and osteoporosis are all linked to diet and exercise. Americans and their children are the most over-fed and under-nourished group of people in the world.

> One out of two Americans is overweight.
> One-third of Americans are obese.
> Being overweight is the second leading cause of preventable death in the U.S.

ILLNESS AND DISEASE IS COSTING AMERICA BIG BUCKS

The total cost of stroke to the United States is estimated at about $43 billion per year.

> $28 billion per year direct costs for medical care and therapy
> $15,000 is the average cost of care for a patient for up to 90 days after a stroke.
> $35,000 for 10% of patients, the cost of care for the first 90 days after a stroke.

*Statistics compiled from the Pennsylvania Health Care Cost Containment Council "Hospital Performance Report: 28 Common Medical Procedures and Treatments" (December 2002)

SALES AND MARKETING STRATEGIES OF THE FOOD AND BEVERAGE INDUSTRY

The food and beverage industry as well as the health and wellness industry have a leadership responsibility to clean up their marketing. Misinformation and misleading claims are rampant. Observe carefully and you will detect the emotion-laden words which are associated with poor choices and portion sizes:

> Convenient (over-processed)
> All natural (so is lard and corn syrup)
> Lite or light (lots of added sugar)

Quick and easy (huge amounts of sodium)
Simple (check the label; not-so-simple, unpronounceable ingredients.)

And the list goes on:

Fun, exciting, easy, time saver, feels great, low-carb, no sugar, no fat, healthy, look great.

Will the food and beverage industry have an economic price to pay for such changes? Yes, the transitional period will have some associated costs, in the short term. In the long run, the food and beverage industry as well as consumers and our country as a whole will all benefit from a healthier America with healthier food choices. In fact, this will result in innovation and new areas of revenue for the food and beverage industry, all while actively contributing to making Americans and America healthier and stronger.

THE PUBLIC'S BASIC RIGHT TO KNOW

Disclosure is the law for government in Florida and many other states and federal entities. The Sunshine Law of Florida establishes a basic right of access to most meetings of boards, commissions and other governing bodies of state and local governmental agencies or authorities. It has led not only to a more informed public, but actually better government.

Full disclosure on food labels would likewise inform the public and result in healthier foods being produced and marketed. True full disclosure for the average consumer must be in the form of a simple "level of healthiness" and "level of nutrients" grade. The factors determining the simple, easy-to-understand grade must be clearly defined in easily understandable language.

HEALTH POLLUTION A NATIONAL SECURITY ISSUE

The present health pollution of America is a national security issue because the consequences go much farther into sociological issues, such as increased crime and poor learning ability. An unhealthy America cannot perform or think as well.

LOOKING FORWARD

Whatever challenges our country faces will be better met if we are healthier in mind and body. Sick and unhealthy Americans are living longer and living with meds. These Americans need to be weaned back to health and off of the meds, where possible. In most cases, lifestyle changes will result in improved health, independent of meds. Our physicians are challenged with a special institutional leadership role in strategizing to prescribe lifestyle-based changes and not just medication so that they truly can take on the role of healers, not only for the patient but also for the nation. Keep America strong. Love America and Americans! The medication mindset without healthy eating and exercise lifestyle changes is killing Americans.

MARCHING ORDERS
INSTITUTIONAL RESPONSIBILITY TO FIX OUR HEALTH CRISIS

1. *Portion sizes: Regulate portion sizes for restaurants to conform to healthy eating.*
2. *Nutritional quality of foods: Regulate the quality of food to conform to healthy eating.*
3. *Regulate soft drinks similar to alcohol: Regulate the removal of all soft drinks from our schools, hospitals and businesses. Replace them with water and flavored water. Allow juices only in 8-oz containers.*
4. *Fit and healthy employees: Mandate keeping employees fit and healthy in our workplaces and as a requirement for health insurance. Implement increased premiums for violators and reduced premiums for those who comply. Get some accountability back into the lives of the insured. Group policies with businesses would require the business to keep their employees fit and healthy since this impacts workplace performance, absenteeism and medical costs.*
5. *Unhealthy vending machine choices: Remove vending machines with unhealthy foods and replace with healthy choices that correspond with established dietary guidelines. Alternatively, the portion sizes of sweets and other empty-calorie snacks need to be significantly reduced to save the health of our fellow Americans.*
6. *Sodium, sugar and fat: Regulate the content of sodium, sugar and fat in foods. It's killing our fellow Americans in staggering numbers.*
7. *Uniform serving sizes: Regulate uniform serving sizes on nutritional labels and incorporate a grade which designates the level of healthiness or unhealthiness and why.*
8. *Label with grade of nutritional value: Clearly designate foods that are processed with a warning label about the reduced nutrients and other unhealthy ingredients and then include a grade for the level of healthiness. Do not allow the "injection" of certain vitamins and minerals raise the grade or level of healthiness in processed foods.*

Chapter Ten

Fitness Goals
and
Progress Measurement

Goals Equal Change

"A prudent person foresees the danger ahead and takes precautions; the simpleton goes blindly on and suffers the consequences." Proverbs 22:3 – Bible, New Living Translation

In order to go from Point A to Point B, you've got to know where Point A is. We will establish your Point A in your fitness journey by measuring and testing. You will measure your:

Body Mass Index (BMI)
Size of your body parts
Cardio, strength and muscle endurance
Height and weight

BODY MASS INDEX (BMI)

Body Mass Index (BMI) is a number calculated from a person's height and weight. BMI provides a reliable indicator of body fatness for most people and is used to screen for weight categories that may lead to health problems. If, however, you are a body-builder or naturally have a big, muscular build, BMI may not work as a reliable indicator of progress. Those with a relatively large, muscular build need to understand that they have the special challenge to maintain their cardio conditioning. Otherwise, they are at a heightened risk for health issues specific to that body type.

INTERPRETATION OF BMI FOR ADULTS

For adults 20 years old and older, BMI is interpreted using standard weight status categories that are the same for all ages and for both men and women. For children and teens, on the other hand, the interpretation of BMI is both age- and sex-specific.

STANDARD BMI WEIGHT STATUS CATEGORIES FOR ADULTS

Below 18.5 is underweight.
18.5 to 24.9 is a healthy weight.
25.0 to 29.9 is overweight.
30.0 and above is obese.

EXAMPLE OF SOMEONE WHO IS 5'9" TALL

124 lbs or less is a BMI below 18.5 and is underweight.
125 lbs to 168 lbs is within a BMI range of 18.5 to 24.9 and is a healthy weight.
169 lbs to 202 lbs is within a BMI range of 25.0 to 29.9 and is overweight.
203 lbs or more is a BMI range of 30.0 or higher and is obese.

Source: Centers for Disease Control and Prevention, CDC, website: www.cdc.gov

LET'S TALK ABOUT BODY FAT

I recommend using BMI to easily get an idea of where you stand with healthy or unhealthy body fat. The body fat percentage categories below are guidelines. If you would like a quick and easy way to calculate your body fat, go to the website www.csgnetwork.com/bodyfatcalc.html. This is designed to give the approximate percentage of body fat, based on weight and waist size as compared to tables published by the American Medical Association. Just enter your present weight and waist size.

The American Council on Exercise has categorized ranges of body fat percentages as follows:

Essential fat
Women 12-15%
Men 2-5%

Athletes
Women 16–20%
Men 6–13%

Fitness
Women 21–24%
Men 14–17%

Acceptable
Women 25–31%
Men 18–25%

Obese
Women 32%+
Men 25%+

Essential fat values are lower than the recommended minimum body fat percentage levels. A small amount of *storage* fat is required to be available as fuel for the body in time of need. It can be dangerous to have *essential* body fat levels as low as depicted on the chart above.

BODY MEASUREMENTS USING A TAILOR'S MEASURING TAPE

A quick and simple way to measure loss of body fat is to take body measurements with a measuring tape every four weeks as a part of your M.O.V.E.™ program (see chapter on M.O.V.E. Weight-loss Program). You will need a buddy to take the measurements for you. Always take body measurements on the right side of your body. We will limit the measurements to the following body parts so that you have some fast and easy indicators of your progress. Also, since you will probably be clothed for these measurements, make sure that you are wearing the same clothing for each of the measurements to ensure an accurate measurement of progress. The measurements should be taken at the same time of day, and not just after a meal or a vigorous exercise session.

NECK CIRCUMFERENCE

Your arms are relaxed at your sides in the standing position, and your neck is relaxed. Measure the smallest circumference of your neck, and note the number of inches.

ARM

Measure the arm circumference with the subject standing upright, shoulders relaxed, and the right arm extended out to the side and parallel to the ground. It is important to be certain that the muscle of the arm is not flexed or tightened, which could yield a larger and inaccurate reading. Your buddy will stand facing your right side. Place the tape around the largest part of the bicep/tricep and measure.

CHEST CIRCUMFERENCE

Your arms are relaxed and at your sides. Your buddy takes the measuring tape under your arms and around your chest where the nipples are. Relax your breathing during this measurement.

ABDOMINAL CIRCUMFERENCE

Measure abdominal circumference against the skin at the belly button. Arms are relaxed at the sides. Take a relaxed exhale and have your buddy take the measurement.

WAIST CIRCUMFERENCE

To measure your waist circumference, place a tape measure around your abdominal region just above your hip bone. Be sure that the tape is firm but not too tight. Slowly exhale and take the measurement.

ILIAC CIRCUMFERENCE

Stand and find where your upper pelvic bones protrude the most; you can feel for them on either side of your waist. Measure the circumference at this point. It could be about two inches below the navel (belly button), but can vary from person to person.

HIP CIRCUMFERENCE

Stand and find the area of your body below your navel where you are the widest. This area can vary greatly from person to person. Wrap the tape measure around your body and take the measurement.

CALF CIRCUMFERENCE

You're in the standing position. Relax your right leg and put your weight on your left leg. Now measure the calf circumference of the right at the widest point.

FITNESS TEST

It's time to test your muscle endurance, cardio and strength. All it takes are three very basic activities, push-ups, crunches or sit-ups and a one-mile run/walk. Use the results as a benchmark. You need the benchmark in order to establish reasonable, attainable goals to shoot for every four weeks of testing. For your kick-start program, test yourself every four weeks for four months. After that, you can test yourself every three months or twice a year. If you notice you're falling back to your old ways of insufficient exercise, the fitness test will let you know and become a wake-up call to get back on track.

CONDUCT THE FITNESS TEST EVENTS IN THIS ORDER

1. Push-ups
2. Crunches or sit-ups
3. One mile run/walk

PUSH-UPS (KNEE OR REGULAR)

The push-up will test the endurance of your chest, shoulders and triceps. Rest is permitted in the up position of the push-up or by raising your rearward anatomy while in the upward push-up position. Only correct push-ups count. You have two minutes to perform as many as you can. You count the completed repetition in the up position.

CRUNCHES OR SIT-UPS

Choose regular crunches or sit-ups for this event. The sit-up measures the endurance of your abdominals and hip-flexor muscles. Perform as many as you can within two minutes. You will notice that time is really of the essence when performing this event. Keep the pace up as fast as you reasonably can. Only correct repetitions count. Resting is permitted only in the "up" position for the sit- up. There is no resting position for crunches; continue performing them until the two minutes are up, or stop prior to the two minutes if too fatigued to continue.

ONE MILE RUN/WALK

The one-mile run/walk is designed to measure your aerobic fitness and leg endurance. If, however, you do not have a measured one-mile distance, pick an approximate distance with clear beginning and ending landmarks, and always use this course for your measurement of progress. Your objective is to complete this event as fast as you reasonably can.

RECORD YOUR SCORES AND ESTABLISH YOUR FOUR-WEEK GOALS

You may need some help with establishing your goals. If you are out of shape and just starting out, you will find that, with consistency, you will make significant progress with all three events.

HOW TO ESTABLISH FITNESS GOALS

Let's say you completed the one-mile run/walk in 11 minutes. I would expect that with your next test, you will complete the mile run within a range of 9 to 10 minutes, shaving off one to two minutes of your time. You will conduct a test every four weeks for at least four months. As your fitness improves the goals will probably not be as great a difference, such a shaving off one to two minutes of your time from the mile run.

U.S. Army Fitness Test Scores for 37 to 41 Year Olds		
	Male	**Female**
Push-ups		
Minimum	34	13
Maximum	73	40
Sit-ups		
Minimum	38	38
Maximum	76	76
Two-mile Run		
Minimum	18:16	22:42
Maximum	13:35	17:00

MARCHING ORDERS – FITNESS GOALS AND PROGRESS MEASUREMENT

- *Test your cardio, strength and endurance at least twice a year.*
- *Calculate your Body Mass Index, as necessary.*
- *When kick-starting a fitness program, test yourself every four weeks, calculate your BMI and weigh yourself.*
- *Have a buddy take your body measurements every four weeks to kick-start your health and fitness program.*
- *Get going now and get it in your calendar!*

He should sweep streets so well that all the host of heaven and earth will pause to say, 'Here lives a great street-sweeper who did his job well.'

- Martin Luther King Jr.

Chapter Eleven

Spiritual "Full Metal Jacket"

Change by Finding Your Purpose

Be a truth seeker and listen to your heart. The Creator of all that is and ever was will speak to your heart if you humble yourself and are willing to listen. - Lt. Col. Bob Weinstein, USAR, (ret.)

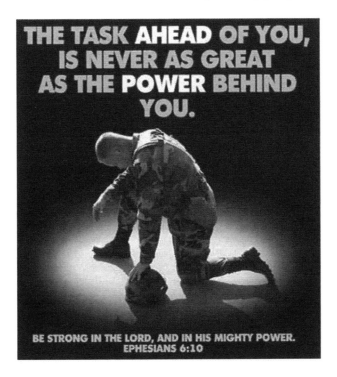

THE TASK **AHEAD OF YOU,** IS NEVER AS GREAT AS THE **POWER BEHIND** YOU.

BE STRONG IN THE LORD, AND IN HIS MIGHTY POWER.
EPHESIANS 6:10

THE RIGHT ATTITUDE IS ESSENTIAL

It is a scientific fact that you will be dead longer than you are alive. A significant part of health that is neglected is a spiritual life. This is a tough topic to tackle with so many views about just what "spiritual" is. I'm going to give you the meat-and-potatoes version. I will also cover some things you may or may not agree with. If you are not ready for some of what I consider to be spiritual truths, skip over it and come back when you are ready. My intent is to encourage thought and not to change you, because YOU are the only one who can change YOU.

Spiritual is not about meditating and praying and going to church *unless* the attitude of your heart is in the right place. Spiritual is about the values discussed at the beginning of this book on the topic of character and Army values. Spiritual is about having an open heart and mind to listen to the Creator. Spiritual is about the humble willingness to recognize that there is right and wrong, good and bad. Spiritual is the willingness to seek out the difference by searching your heart. Spiritual is seeking out the ultimate purpose of life and living. Spiritual is to forgive. My most important relationship is with the Creator and that makes my spiritual life most important since it addresses my underlying purpose for being here.

WHAT IS A SPIRITUAL ATTITUDE? THIS PASSAGE FROM THE BIBLE SUMS IT UP

"Don't be selfish; don't live to make a good impression on others. Be humble, thinking of others as better than yourself. Don't think only about your own affairs, but be interested in others, too, and what they are doing." - Source: Philippians, Chapter 2, vs. 3 - 4, Holy Bible, New Living Translation

THE GOLDEN RULE

The highest law that fulfills all natural laws is the Golden Rule. Jesus Christ was asked the most important question about leading a spiritual life:

"Teacher, which is the most important commandment in the Law of Moses?" Jesus replied, "You must love the Lord with all your heart, all your soul, and all your mind." This is the first and greatest commandment. A second is equally important: 'Love your neighbor as yourself.' - Source: Matthew, Chapter 22, v. 36, Holy Bible, New Living Translation

Your neighbor is everyone else, not just the person next door.

LOVE YOUR ENEMY

Jesus radicalized the Golden Rule:

"You have heard that the Law of Moses says, 'Love your neighbor' and hate your enemy. But I say, love your enemies! Pray for those who persecute you! In that way, you will be acting as true children of your Father in heaven. - Source: Matthew, Chapter 5, v. 43, Holy Bible, New Living Translation

And King Solomon said:

"If your enemies are hungry, give them food to eat. If they are thirsty, give them water to drink." - Source: Proverbs 25: 21-22, Holy Bible, New Living Translation

Love those who are your enemy or are against you in any way or who don't share your view of the world, and you are taking the Golden Rule to its highest level. You will be blessed. Such deeds do not go unnoticed by the Creator.

HATE KILLS, LITERALLY

The opposite of love is hate and hate kills. It "kills" the person with hate in his or her heart. It kills others and is the catalyst for killing both in connection with a faith and when it is secular-based. Any political policy of any nation that promotes hate is wrong. Hate also hurts. It hurts the hater and the "hatee." It makes no difference whether it's opposing religions, opposing political parties, different nationalities, opposing countries or opposing individuals in society or a family. In this time of election campaigns, all parties and candidates need to be respectful in dealing with each other while addressing the issues they consider important.
        This applies to the media as well. The personal attacks and hate language need to stop.

THERE ARE MANY RELIGIONS

There are many religions, some similar, most different. Many will embrace the universal values that have been embedded in our hearts by the Creator. Which one is the right one? All of them? Some of them or just one? Ask God, the Creator of all that is. If you have an open and humble heart and are truly seeking the truth, the Creator will find you. The Golden Rule and the radicalized form of loving your neighbor and your enemy are natural laws endowed by the Creator. Violation of them will have consequences spiritually as well as from the standpoint of health and wellness.

SHARK-INFESTED WATERS

By now, some of you may very well be questioning who the Creator is. Do you really want to find out? Many soldiers in the South Pacific during the Second World War found a quick answer to the question of who the Creator is. They found themselves in shark-infested waters clinging together with arms interlocked. Occasionally a shark would attack and devour one of them. There were no dogma discussions about religion. They prayed and they prayed together and they prayed with all of their hearts and souls. To whom did they all pray? What attitude did they have? Were they humble?

THE DECISION MAKER

These soldiers swimming in the shark-infested waters knew to whom they were praying. No one had to tell them. They were praying to the one in charge of all of creation. They were praying to the decision maker. They knew that if they could reach the decision maker of all that is, they would have hope. There were no philosophical discussions about the value of prayer. They knew it was the only way to communicate with the Creator of all that is. How did they know that? That is the question I would like you to think about.

If you're interested in following a true story from the perspective of one of the soldiers in the South Pacific during the Second World War, I recommend the book by David Harrell, as told by Edgar Harrell, USMC, "Out of the Depths," a survivor's story of the sinking of the USS Indianapolis.

DO YOU NEED A CRISIS TO BE HUMBLE?

Will you need a crisis situation of life or death to humble your heart and seek out the decision maker of all that is? Hopefully not. I don't wish the situation of those South Pacific soldiers on anyone. You will be dead longer than you are alive. You might as well give it a shot at getting to know the Creator before you check-in. You've got nothing to lose and much to gain by doing so.

THE CONFLICT NEVER ENDS

The conflict never ends because the real conflict is within, even when leading a spiritual life. To disregard this important truth will make you vulnerable.

RELATIONSHIP IS KEY

You might want to be greeted at check in time with "How are you?" instead of "Who are you?" by the Creator. As with all relationships, communication and time spent together is necessary. It's no different with the Creator. After all, the Creator is the decision maker and the Maker even though sometimes it doesn't seem to be the case from our human perspective and with our limited intellect.

IN SALES, THE DECISION MAKER IS KEY

Ask any salesperson desiring to sell products and services who they want to talk with in order to have a shot at making the sale. It is the decision maker. And good salespeople will always ask who the decision maker is when discussing potential business with a company or potential client. You need to do the same when it comes to the Creator, and that requires a certain humbled and open attitude of the heart to be successful in your spiritual quest. You may have heard the very applicable expression, "When the student is ready, the teacher appears." I can attest to that. If you take this journey, you will not be disappointed.

"FULL METAL JACKET" – NOT EVERYONE IS READY FOR THIS

This last segment on the topic of a spiritual life is for those who are looking for the "Full Metal Jacket" experience. "Full Metal Jacket" means there's more to a spiritual life than "just" being good. Is it sufficient to maintain the relationship with the Creator when you die and report in to "Higher Headquarters" simply by leading a good life? Can we earn salvation granting eternal fellowship with the Creator? Some of you may be thinking at this point. "Salvation? What for? I'm a good person." Well, have you ever lied or stolen something or thought thoughts about others that were less then honorable? I think your answer to this question is probably "Yes." I am going to make the bold assumption that no one can answer this question with a "No." I sure can't.

Truth is unshakable and independent of how we perceive it, ignore it, reject it or accept it. I have wandered both close and far from the spiritual truth about salvation and a relationship with the Creator of all that is. I have gone through many changes in my life. When I returned from Berlin, Germany back in 1995, I was determined to seek and improve my life by working on my character and understanding that I am the only one who can change me. This improvement journey and desire to find my ultimate purpose led me to the understanding that I am a sinner and that I, on my own, cannot extract this inclination to sin that is inside of me. I sought through prayer and study a relationship with the Creator and Jesus Christ. I accepted his authority, asked Him to accompany me every day of my life and I asked for forgiveness of my sins. Most importantly, I have the certainty that I will not live (after death) in eternal separation from God. I was created to be with Him and I want to return to where I belong.

GOOD DEEDS NOT ENOUGH

Recently, I experienced an amazing story of compassion that broke all the societal rules as we know them. My brother, Bill, agreed to take in and care for the terminally ill former husband of his wife. He had cancer, had only three months to live and had no other family members to take care of him. He passed away at Bill's home with Bill and his wife to comfort him. At the funeral, the story about Bill caring for him was greeted with astonishment. The funeral director had lots of stories about families who did not talk to one another and he was delighted and impressed by such a demonstration of love and compassion. And still, good deeds are not enough ...

EVERYONE, WITHOUT EXCEPTION, HAS VIOLATED MORAL LAWS

I am also going to make the bold statement that we are all sinners and that includes me. If you answered "Yes" to the above question about ever telling a lie or stealing or thinking less then honorable thoughts about someone else you have violated moral laws. Sin is the violation of moral laws. That makes us all sinners since we all, at sometime, and possibly every day, have violated moral laws, at least in our attitudes towards others.

I am going to make a further bold statement; it is a violation of moral laws not to love yourself and treat yourself in a respectful manner like you would a very best friend. The only one I have found who has been authorized to grant the "Full Metal Jacket" or salvation, granting fellowship with the Creator after death, is Jesus Christ. This is a faith decision and is between you and the Creator and that is something you will have to take up with Him, if you are not ready to accept this (or are ready). In order to grant anything, one must first have the authority to do so. I believe He has that authority.

Some of you might be thinking about some of the bad church experiences or some of the bad things that have happened in church history. That's nothing new. Read the scriptures carefully and you will find many instances of bad behavior. Don't let that influence your personal relationship with the Creator.

Whether you have accepted this offer by the Creator through Jesus Christ or not, no good deed (or bad one) goes unnoticed. Such salvation is not a "license" to do what we want. The Golden Rule makes that very clear as to how ourrelationship with the Creator, our fellow man and woman, and ourselves should be. For those who need more food for thought, I recommend the book by *C. S. Lewis, "Mere Christianity."* The contents of the book stem from a radio talk by C. S. Lewis between 1942 and 1944. C. S. Lewis is described as one of theintellectual giants of the twentieth century. He was an atheist and describes in his book how this changed in his life.

FORGIVENESS AND FORGIVING

So how can we possibly stand before the Creator, if we are not able to meet His high standards? That's where forgiveness comes in. Ask for the Creator's forgiveness and don't forget to forgive yourself and others. Forgiveness is a part of the Golden Rule. There are no exceptions when it comes to forgiving others and yourself. Bitterness or lack of forgiveness is like drinking poison and expecting the other person to die. We are to hold no grudge towards anyone. If you do, your health and your spiritual life will suffer and you will be causing harm to others.

BENEFITS OF A SPIRITUAL LIFE

Leading a spiritual life will positively impact your health and you will be happier.

You will be more thankful and appreciative of life and others.
You will sleep better.
You will have less stress.
You will deal with conflicts with patience and calm.
You will forgive bad behavior.
Your discernment of right and wrong will improve.

You will have less worry.

You will be more disciplined and focused on what is more important.

You will have greater wisdom.

You will make more friends.

You will be kind to yourself.

You will value yourself and others.

You will cease to make excuses.

You will be a better friend.

You will pray.

Chapter Twelve

Real Weight-loss Successes

Real People Change
You Can Too

"Life is a self-fulfilling prophesy. You may not always get what you want, but in the long run you will get what you expect." - Denis Waitley

HOW MIKKI LOST 65 POUNDS

FROM DRESS SIZE 16 TO 4

Mikki Schroeder has been attending my Beach Boot Camp group classes on Fort Lauderdale Beach for the past couple of years. She is 33
years old and did not really begin her weight-loss and exercise journey until the age of 32. She is an office manager/executive assistant and has a sedentary job. At 5'4' tall, her present weight is 136 pounds. She weighed 110 pounds in high school. Before she started her successful weight-loss program at the age of 32, Mikki weighed 201 pounds. She has lost 65 pounds of excess weight. She went from a dress size of 16 to her present size 4. Her BMI or 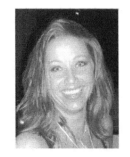 Body Mass Index when she weighed 201 pounds was 34.4 which is obese on the BMI scale. Her present BMI weighing in at 136 pounds results in a BMI of 23.4 which puts her in the healthy range.

Mikki will share in her own words how she took back control of her health and lifestyle.

Colonel Bob: What lessons have you learned on your weight-loss journey?

Mikki: Start now! Don't wait until Monday or whatever day. Never call it a diet. It's a change in how you live your life. Try new things. You don't have to go to the gym to get exercise. There is no quick fix or miracle cure. You didn't gain weight overnight; you're not going to lose it overnight either.

Colonel Bob: What were some of the phases of weight and eating habits you went through?

Mikki: When I first started, I only changed how and what I ate. I didn't really change my exercise habits or lack thereof. I did lose weight; however I wasn't getting the results from my body that I wanted. I still didn't have any energy, I still lost my breath quickly, and my body parts (ladies, you know the ones) still jiggled. I knew that I had to incorporate regular exercise into my life. Once I did that, my health started to improve greatly.

Colonel Bob: What were your greatest challenges and how did you overcome them?

Mikki: Since I always ate what I want, when I wanted it, my biggest challenge was changing the way I ate. I chose to join Weight Watchers in order to teach myself healthy eating habits. The main thing Weight Watchers taught me was portion control. Also, it's not about deprivation, it's about moderation. It's OK to allow yourself treats occasionally. Weight Watchers also taught me to be aware of the nutritional values. I now read the labels on everything.

Another challenge was maintaining a regular exercise routine. When I first started exercising again, I got tired very easily, couldn't keep up, felt weak and nauseated. It would have been very easy to give up and say I just can't do it. I had to make a real conscious effort to push forward and continue, knowing that things would get better.

Colonel Bob: What keeps you on track?

Mikki: The way I look and more importantly the way I feel keep me on track. The difference in the way I feel now compared to when I was overweight is astounding. There is no comparison!

Not only did I see the results on the scale, but I saw them in my body. Every couple of weeks I had to buy new clothes or have old ones taken in. Sometimes before I even had a chance to wear something that I just bought, it was already too big.

Colonel Bob: What is your weight history starting from high school?

Mikki: Growing up, I was always thin and weighed between 98 and 110 pounds in high school. I didn't play sports but was very active with dance and could always eat whatever I wanted to. That also meant I ate the quantity I wanted and as often as I wanted. In my early 20's, I found out I had a condition called hypo-thyroidism, which is an underactive thyroid. Since the main function of the thyroid is to control your metabolism, and mine wasn't, slowly but surely, I started to gain weight.

Colonel Bob: What changes have you made in your eating habits?

Mikki: The biggest change I made was portion control. I have also incorporated more fruits, vegetables and whole grains. I am very careful in watching my sugar and fat intake. It's all about moderation, not deprivation. If I want a piece of chocolate cake, I have a piece; a small piece, not the whole cake and not every day.

Colonel Bob: Did you use a support system or was someone else there to support and encourage you?

Mikki: The reactions and encouragement I received from my family and friends was all the support I needed, especially when those around you get motivated to improve their own health.

Colonel Bob: How do you see your health over the next five, ten and twenty years and how can you impact on your health over the long-term?

Mikki: I see my health continuing to improve throughout the years. There is no way I will allow myself to fall back into bad habits. What I am doing now will ward off many health issues/problems that people experience as they get older.

Colonel Bob: Have you or do you have set-backs and how do you or have you overcome them?

Mikki: I have been very fortunate in that I haven't had any set-backs. When I started my life change, I made up my mind that no matter what, I was going to remain positive and continue to eat right and exercise. I was not going to allow myself to slip back into the bad habit of emotional eating.

Throughout this process, I have not gained any weight back. When I had periods of no weight-loss, I took a look at what I was eating to be sure I was staying on track. I continued to exercise and eat right. Even though I wasn't losing weight, I still saw results in my body, losing inches and gaining muscle.

However, I have had periods of no weight-loss even though I was eating right and exercising regularly. I think so many of us, especially women, get discouraged when we know we are doing what we should and we don't think we are getting the results we want. Because of my mindset, I realized that it was not just about losing weight, it was about getting healthy. And because I knew I was doing what I should, I was getting results, my body was becoming healthier.

HOW GREG LOST 60 POUNDS
FROM PANT SIZE 44 TO 33

Greg Gregory has been attending my Beach Boot Camp personal training on Fort Lauderdale Beach for three years now. He is 42 years old and did not really begin his exercise and weight-loss journey until the age of 39. Fifteen years of gradual weight gain took him from his high school weight of 190 pounds all the way up to 262. He is self- employed, travels a lot and has a predominantly sedentary job. At 6'4", his present weight is 202 pounds. Greg gradually lost 60 pounds over the 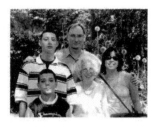 three years of regular exercise and making eating adjustments along the way. He went from a pant size of 44 to his present size 33. His BMI or Body Mass Index when he weighed 262 pounds was 31.9, which classified him as obese. His present BMI is 24.6 puts him right in the healthy range. Greg will share with you how he took back control of his health and lifestyle.

Colonel Bob: What lessons have you learned on your weight-loss journey?

Greg: It's all about attitude. It's about creating focus and determination. It's about making gradual adjustments along the way until it becomes a healthy lifestyle. I realized that getting older doesn't have to mean getting less active. What I have noticed is the significant impact it has had on my improved health and increased energy.

Colonel Bob: What were some of the phases of weight and eating habits you went through?

Greg: The first phase was fighting the battle of the bad habits and sticking with it. I made changes in my eating habits from unhealthy to healthier choices and I also reduced the quantity of food I was eating to put it in balance with my weight-loss and exercise program. Once I lost the weight, the key was to balance eating and exercise with the weight I wanted to maintain.

Colonel Bob: What were your greatest challenges and how did you overcome them?

Greg: I first needed to recognize that I needed to get started. My present lifestyle without exercise and a healthy weight had to change since my health is of utmost importance. The best thing I did to get me on the right track was to put it in my calendar and treat it like any business meeting. I had to be there.

Colonel Bob: What keeps you on track?

Greg: My relationship with God keeps me on track. I started this relationship in 2001.

Colonel Bob: What is your weight history starting from high school?

Greg: During my high school and college years my weight was between 185 and 210. When I weighed 210 in college that was muscle gain and not fat. After college my weight started to gradually increase over a period of 15 years, from the age of 25 to 40. I ended up tipping the scales with 260 pounds and that was not muscle gain. It was fat.

Colonel Bob: What changes have you made in your eating habits?

Greg: I started eating breakfast. I stopped drinking sodas. I drank my coffee without sugar and used a non-dairy soy creamer. I reduced bread in my diet. I reduced cheese. For many years my cholesterol was high and my doctor was about to prescribe medication. I experimented by eliminating cheese and dairy products from my diet for 30 days and my cholesterol dropped without medication. I am eating more fish and less red meat. I no longer eat big late-night meals. If I have to eat late, I will eat a small meal.

Colonel Bob: Did you use a support system or was someone else there to support and encourage you?

Greg: Yes. I used a support system. I sought advice on healthy eating and I continue to train with you. Accountability and encouragement have played an important role.

Colonel Bob: How do you see your health over the next five, ten and twenty years and how can you impact on your health over the long-term?

Greg: Continue with the healthy lifestyle I have achieved. Set positive challenges and goals along the way to keep me on track. In high school and college I was active. I now seek out recreational activities, such as biking, hiking and basketball. Staying active is key.

Colonel Bob: Have you or do you have set-backs and how do you or have you overcome them?

Greg: Yes. Every now and then I find myself wandering off eating a little too much of the foods I shouldn't or eating too much. I make sure that these remain temporary set-backs and do not become permanent. This is also where a system of accountability is important. My family helps me to overcome any set-backs that may occur.

How Priscilla Lost 38 Pounds
From Dress Size 14 To 6

Priscilla Smith has been attending my Beach Boot Camp group classes on Fort Lauderdale Beach for the past couple of years. She is 55 years old and did not really begin her weight-loss journey until the age of 51 and an exercise program at the age of 53. She is a court reporter and has a predominantly sedentary job. At 5'6' tall, her present weight is 130 pounds. She weighed 125 pounds in high school. Before she started her successful weight-loss program at the age of 51, Priscilla weighed 168 pounds. She has lost 38 pounds of excess weight. She went from a dress size of 14 to her present size 6. Her BMI or Body Mass Index when she weighed 168 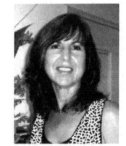 pounds was 28.8 which classified her as overweight on the BMI scale. Her present BMI is 21 which puts her right in the middle of the healthy range. Priscilla will share in her own words how she took back control of her health and lifestyle.

Colonel Bob: What lessons have you learned on your weight-loss journey?

Priscilla: A successful weight-loss eating plan has to reduce, not increase, my hunger. I eliminate the "wrong" foods -- sugar in all its forms (high-fructose corn syrup, molasses, and honey) and eat plant products with low sugar and high fiber -- to lose weight. Reading about physiology and diet theories was necessary for me to understand my body's reaction to different foods and to find motivation.

It's what and how much I eat, not why, how, or when I eat that determines gain or loss. Any excuse or negative attitude can become, instead, a motivation and reason to improve. "I have a slow metabolism, so I can't lose weight" becomes "I have a slow metabolism, so it's all the more important that I lose weight."

Colonel Bob: What were some of the phases of weight and eating habits you went through?

Priscilla: I was always on the normal-to-slightly-heavy side. Because traditional diets -- counting calories, or fat grams, or following the food pyramid -- were ineffective, I followed a random pattern of weight-loss and gain until I was over 40 and ready to make another life change.

Colonel Bob: What were your greatest challenges and how did you overcome them?

Priscilla: Obsessing over food planning and preparation and constant hunger made losing weight difficult. I could overcome these by selecting the right foods, by reading nutrition labels for one thing only -- grams of sugar -- and reading ingredient labels to avoid anything unpronounceable. When I switched to "caveman foods;" that is, food that was available to our ancestors, planning became simple, and the simple foods eliminated my hunger.

Colonel Bob: What keeps you on track?

Priscilla: Reading about physiology helps to motivate me. I use a fat-percentage bathroom scale. My numbers (cholesterol, etc.) are improving, so not only am I losing weight, but my tissues and organs are getting healthier and flourishing rather than deteriorating and aging, which is my real goal here.

Colonel Bob: What is your weight history starting from high school?

Priscilla: I weighed 125 pounds in high school. I was healthy. I wasn't overweight till college. The dorm had an all-you-can-eat buffet three meals a day with Southern food I wasn't exposed to as a kid. I slowly gained again. Over the years, I gained to the point of weighing 168 pounds at the age of 51. I lost 38 pounds over a period of a couple of years. My present weight is 130 pounds. That's going from a dress size of 14 to a 6.

Colonel Bob: What changes have you made in your eating habits?

Priscilla: I try to upgrade every food choice. To illustrate, I don't drink orange juice anymore (too many grams of sugar) but an occasional orange is an upgrade (more fiber). I upgrade my beverage to water or green tea without sugar.

Colonel Bob: Did you use a support system or was someone else there to support and encourage you?

Priscilla: I didn't use a support system for losing weight. I just kept from being misled by product claims, for example, and I read, read, read those books and food nutrition labels.

Colonel Bob: How do you see your health over the next five, ten and twenty years and how can you impact on your health over the long-term?

Priscilla: The next half of my life will be healthier than the first. I have increased my longevity. That means I will have more time to "get it right"! We're all running towards a cliff; by losing weight, I've slowed down my pace.

Colonel Bob: Have you or do you have set-backs and how do you or have you overcome them?

Priscilla: Traveling, holidays, and other upsets of the daily routine set me back sometimes. I compensate by devoting more to my exercise regimen or adding a challenging wrinkle to it. That gets me back on track more quickly. I use self-talk. When offered or facing a bad food choice, I say aloud or to myself, "I don't eat those anymore."

How Lou Lost 29 Pounds
From Pant Size 46 To 40

Lou Taylor has been attending my Beach Boot Camp personal training on Fort Lauderdale Beach for several months. He is 55 years old and did not really begin his exercise and weight-loss journey until the age of 51. At 6' 3", his present weight is 260 pounds. He weighed 125 pounds in high school and was an avid swimmer. Before he started his weight-loss program at the age of 54, he weighed 291 pounds. He has so far lost 29 pounds of excess weight. He went from a pant size of 46 to his present Size 40. His BMI or Body Mass Index when he weighed 291 pounds was 36.3 which classified him as obese. His present BMI of 32.5 is still in the obese range. He has had 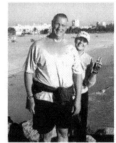 onset diabetes and he knows that diabetes is very dangerous so he's working on getting back to a healthy weight and healthy lifestyle. Lou will share with you how he is taking back control of his health and lifestyle.

Colonel Bob: What lessons have you learned on your weight-loss journey?

Lou: You have to work harder at it when you get older. You have to know what you want and what is bad for you. You have to change your way of thinking to recreate your lifestyle so that it reflects the health that you truly want as you get older.

Colonel Bob: What were your greatest challenges and how did you overcome them?

Lou: The biggest struggle has been portion control. The other challenge has been to become more aware of eating quality foods and reducing fats and sugars. It has been challenging for me to push away from a plate of food when I have had enough to eat. I still have the Depression-Era mentality of cleaning my plate no matter how much food is on it. It didn't matter whether I was still hungry or not. I had to clean it. I'm still struggling with this one. How I overcome this one is to make sure not too much food ends up on my plate and, if it does, to stop eating when I have had enough.

Colonel Bob: What keeps you on track?

Lou: My wife, Trudie has been great support for me. She joined Jenny Craig with me to help with the portion sizes and she joins me to train with you.

Colonel Bob: What is your weight history starting from high school?

Lou: I weighed 125 pounds in high school and was an avid swimmer. After high school things went down hill. I had little or no exercise regimen during my working years and watched my weight constantly increase until I reached 291 pounds. At the age of 54, I decided I had to change my lifestyle so that I can age with good health, have more energy and enjoy life more. I am now down to 260 pounds as a 55-year-old, and am working on losing more weight, since my BMI of 32.5 is still in the obese range.

Colonel Bob: What changes have you made in your eating habits?

Lou: My wife and I joined Jenny Craig to help us learn portion control and lose the excess weight. The changes I need to make are to cut out pasta, bread, cheese and red meat from my diet, since they are significant sources of high calories, fat and bad carbs. The red meat and cheese are high sources of cholesterol and fat. We eat out a lot, so we really need to strategize in advance about how we will take control of the menu and design a healthy meal. Desserts are off the menu except for once a week.

Colonel Bob: How do you see your health over the next five, ten and twenty years and how can you impact on your health over the long-term?

Lou: Continue to pursue a healthy lifestyle until it becomes a part of my life. Since my BMI is still in the obese range, my strategy is to break the weight-loss down into phases.

> Phase I: Achieve a weight of 220 – 230 lbs, BMI 27.5 to 28.7 (overweight range)
>
> Phase II: Achieve a weight of 206 – 210 lbs, BMI 25.8 to 26.3 (overweight range)
>
> Phase III: Achieve a weight of 195 – 205 lbs, BMI 24.4 – 25.7 (healthy – overweight range)

I want to stay on a healthy eating plan and eat out no more than once a week and keep up my exercise regimen of three to five times per week.

Colonel Bob: Have you or do you have set-backs, and how do you or have you overcome them?

Lou: Yes. I overcome them by making a pact with my wife, Trudie, to get back on track. The key for me is to make sure the set-backs are only temporary and not permanent. I just get my exercise regimen back into my calendar and then show up and get it done. I use the same approach to get myself back on track with healthy eating, proper portion sizes and reduced sugar and fat. I treat eating and exercise just like a business project that must be accomplished. No ifs, ands or buts.

How Trudie Lost 23 Pounds
From Dress Size 12 To 8

Trudie Taylor has been attending my Beach Boot Camp personal training and group classes on Fort Lauderdale Beach for the past several months. She is 52 years old and has spent her life since high school yo-yo dieting with every imaginable weight-loss diet on the market. In her early 40's she did achieve a weight of 127 pounds but she did not keep it off. At 5'5 ½" tall, she eventually gained to the point of weighing 177 pounds at the age of 52. She weighed 145 pounds in high school. After starting her lifestyle based exercise and healthy eating regimen 3 months ago, she has gone from 177 pounds to her present weight of 154 pounds. She has lost 23 pounds of excess weight. She went from a dress size of 12 to her present 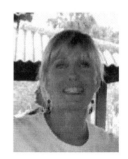 size 8. Her BMI or Body Mass Index when she weighed 177 pounds was 28.6 which is obese on the BMI scale. Her present BMI weighing in at 154 pounds results in a BMI of 24.8 which puts her in the healthy range. Trudie will share in her own words how she took back control of her health and lifestyle.

Colonel Bob: What lessons have you learned on your weight-loss journey?

Trudie: Many. It's hard work and dedication. Never give up since my health is most important to me. I have learned about my limitations and to accept my body as it is so that I don't create any of that unhealthy view of not liking myself regardless of my weight. I need to fully accept and like myself as I am while also working on improving my health through exercise and proper eating. I know that is the healthy approach to improving how I look. How I look is no longer determined by some marketing gimmick or magazine cover look.

Colonel Bob: What were some of the phases of weight and eating habits you went through?

Trudie: I would binge on sugar and sweets. I have always exercised. All that yo-yo dieting was a deviation from back-to-basics living of simply balancing healthy eating with exercise. I am now focusing on back-to-basics eating and exercising.

Colonel Bob: What were your greatest challenges, and how did you overcome them?

Trudie: My greatest challenge was not listening to some of the negative input I received from others which had an unhealthy impact on my self-image of how I looked. I experienced an unhealthy attitude towards my weight. I now understand, regardless of my weight and appearance that I always think good thoughts about myself and value myself as I should while pursuing improvement in a healthy weight and healthy life. This has helped me to enjoy life's journey much more and to enjoy those lifestyle changes on the road to optimal health.

Colonel Bob: What keeps you on track?

Trudie: I want the weight-loss for me, because I want to be healthy, not because some TV advertisement or someone else is pressuring me to change my appearance.

Colonel Bob: What is your weight history starting from high school?

Trudie: I weighed 145 pounds in high school. I am now 52 years old and have spent my life since high school yo-yo dieting with every imaginable weight- loss diet on the market. In my early 40's I did achieve a weight of 127 pounds but did not keep it off. At 5'5 ½" tall, I eventually gained to the point of weighing 177 pounds at the age of 52. After starting my lifestyle-based exercise and healthy eating regimen three months ago, I have gone from 177 pounds to my present weight of 154. I have lost 23 pounds of excess weight. I went from a dress size of 12 to my present Size 8.

Colonel Bob: What changes have you made in your eating habits?

Trudie: No more crazy dieting. I am now back-to-basics of watching the quantity and quality of food I eat. I have realized that the lifestyle-based way of maintaining my health is also the way to look and feel great.

Colonel Bob: Did you use a support system or was someone else there to support and encourage you?

Trudie: Yes. I used a support system which continues on my healthy lifestyle journey. I received support from some of the diet centers and from my family. Training with you has also helped me get back to a healthy lifestyle.

Colonel Bob: How do you see your health over the next five, ten and twenty years and how can you impact on your health over the long-term?

Trudie: I see my health being excellent over many years to come with healthy, enjoyable eating and exercising.

Colonel Bob: Have you or do you have set-backs and how do you or have you overcome them?

Trudie: Yes. There are struggles and conflicts within me. I have been a sugar addict and remain vigilant so that any deviation from healthy eating is only temporary. That's when I take charge and take back control.

HOW SARAH LOST 23 POUNDS
FROM DRESS SIZE 20 TO 16

Sarah Olsen has been attending my Beach Boot Camp group classes on Fort Lauderdale Beach for the past couple of months. She is 24 years old and is 5'9" tall. She started her lifestyle based weight-loss/exercise program at the age of 23 when she weighed 269 pounds. In high school she weighed as much as 175 pounds and graduated at 140 pounds. After starting her lifestyle based exercise and healthy eating regimen about six weeks ago, she has gone from 269 pounds to her present weight of 238 pounds. She has so far lost 31 pounds of excess weight. She went from a dress size of 20 to her present Size 16. Her BMI or Body Mass Index when she weighed 269 pounds was over 40.5, which is obese on the BMI scale. Her present BMI, weighing in at 238 pounds, results in 35.1, which still puts her in the obese range, and is a significant improvement following her healthy, gradual weight-loss approach. Sarah will share in her own words how she is taking back control of her health and lifestyle.

Colonel Bob: What lessons have you learned on your weight-loss journey?

Sarah: That it takes time, patience and a willingness to love who you are right now, no matter what. It's not okay to be ashamed of what you look like and give up. You have to give it everything you have; otherwise, you won't know what you're capable of.

Colonel Bob: What were some of the phases of weight and eating habits you went through?

Sarah: In high school I developed an eating disorder, so I mastered the art of becoming thin quickly. Of course, my eating habits were horrific, consisting mostly of celery with mustard, lettuce, tomato. I knew what the calorie and fat count was of just about everything. The poor eating habits stayed with me until 2004, when it became life or death. Once I decided to get healthy, I started overeating, which isn't uncommon in people with eating disorders - to go one way and then the opposite. When I got promoted at work, I decided I needed to get truly healthy so I can be proud of every part of me.

Colonel Bob: What were your greatest challenges, and how did you overcome them?

Sarah: Old habits die hard; and knowing eating disorders so intimately, my instincts kicked in almost immediately after I made the decision to get healthy the smart way. So far it's been tough, and I can't say it's been a perfect journey, but the commitment I've made to get heart-healthy instead of focusing on the weight usually wins over the desire to make it happen quickly. If I feel like going back, then I try and take a walk or spend time with someone else so it's more difficult to make an unhealthy decision.

Colonel Bob: What keeps you on track?

Sarah: Knowing that at the end of the day I will be able to look back and know I did it with my will power and strength, along with the support of my loved ones. Not only will I be able to say I didn't take the easy road, but I'll have discovered new pieces of myself.

Colonel Bob: What is your weight history starting from high school?

Sarah: Since I moved to America, most of my activities stopped and I began to gain weight. I became more and more secluded and the availability of junk food was astounding. As I realized I hated the outer version of myself with my weight of 175, I tried everything to lose the pounds. Quickly I discovered an easy way to do it and began to drop the weight instantly, it literally took three months to go from a Size 14 to a 6, and that was in high school. I have gone up and down for the past six years, since graduating, always returning to the same method to lose. My intent now is to focus on both healthy eating and regular exercise.

Colonel Bob: What changes have you made in your eating habits?

Sarah: I read a lot about proper eating, and decided the best thing would be for me to turn vegetarian. I'm on the road to becoming vegan; I'm just not there yet. It's definitely helped cut out a lot of the junk.

Colonel Bob: Did you use a support system or was someone else there to support and encourage you?

Sarah: Yes. This time is the first time I've had someone to support and encourage me. My husband is fantastic at encouraging me to go and work out and eat properly. I am eternally grateful for his support.

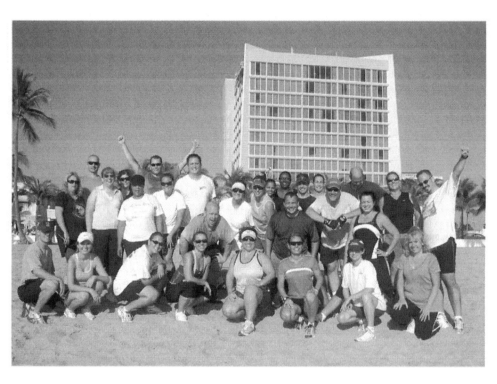

Col. Bob's Beach Boot Camp Class, Fort Lauderdale, FL

PART TWO

THE EXERCISES

The definition of insanity is doing the same thing over and over again and expecting a different result.

- Albert Einstein

Chapter Thirteen

Complete Body Stretch

Stretches

There are many views about stretching and its benefits. If done properly, stretching can be a relaxing and stress relieving experience. Some say that we should stretch before exercising. Others say we should stretch after exercising and still others emphasize stretching before and after. There is no substantial evidence about the benefits of stretching as it pertains to exercise or that it helps prevent injury. If you are involved in high-impact sports or athletic activity requiring the use of lots of agility, stretching could result in creating instability and actually result in injury.

My main concern is too much precious time is spent focusing on stretching and thereby neglecting the cardio and strength training which is a higher priority. Performing all movement exercises, be it strength training or cardio, results in promoting flexibility.

Stretch briefly between exercises. Please remember that you may want to leave stretching out altogether from time to time when performing a circuit routine that combines the cardio and strength training, because you want to maximize the cardio and muscle endurance benefit.

NECK

The neck is such a neglected body part when it comes to exercise. The head spends most of its time just being attached to the neck with little movement except for the guys who suddenly gain extraordinary neck movement capability when the opposite sex happens to be passing by. You just might save a trip to the chiropractor if you exercise the neck on a regular basis and you will promote neck mobility as you age.

Standing or lying down on your back, you will be moving your neck left to right and nodding forward and back. Let's start off with left to right. Whilelooking straight ahead, attempt to touch your right ear to your right shoulder and then your left ear to your left shoulder. The object is to keep your head facing straight ahead and not tilting to the left or right while performing the exercise. Do five to ten repetitions, depending on how your neck feels. Now you're going to nod forward and then back. Use a smooth motion for these neck exercises. Nod forward with your chin to your chest and then lift your head back as far as you comfortably can to look skyward (if standing). Do five to ten reps always using a smooth motion with no jerking.

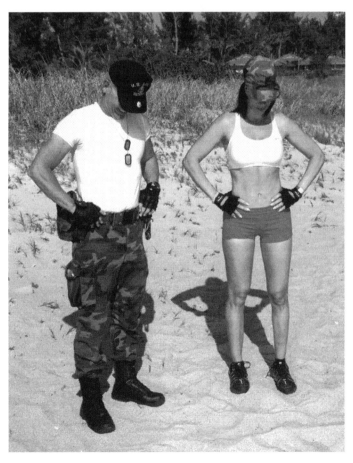

ARMS AND SHOULDERS

Take your right arm and place it across your chest parallel to the ground. With your left hand, reach over and grab your right elbow. Now gently pull your right arm across your chest with your left hand. Hold for 15 to 20 seconds. Switch arms and perform the same stretch.

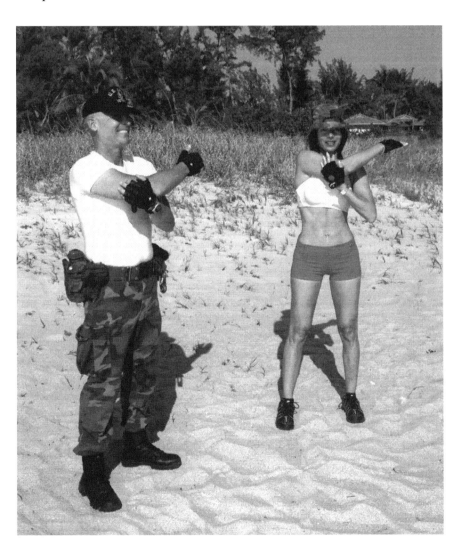

ARM ROTATIONS

This next stretch is actually a great way to work the shoulder muscles and a great warm-up exercise. Now extend your arms out to the sides parallel to the ground like you're going to fly with palms facing down. Rotate in a big circle, first forward for 20 seconds and then reverse. For great shoulder work, just continue to rotate those arms until fatigue starts kicking in while randomly alternating between forward and reverse rotations. You will eventually feel the shoulders burn. Then go back and do the arms and shoulders stretch.

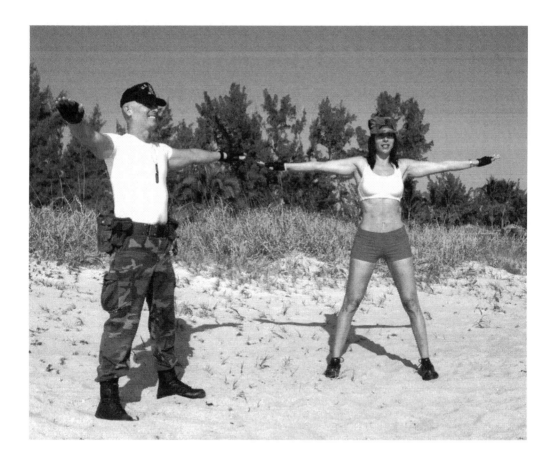

CHEST STRETCH

In the standing position with feet shoulder-width apart, extend your arms out to the sides and parallel to the ground. Slowly pull your arms back as far as you comfortably can. Hold for 20 seconds. This will prepare you for my most favorite exercises, such as push-ups and dips.

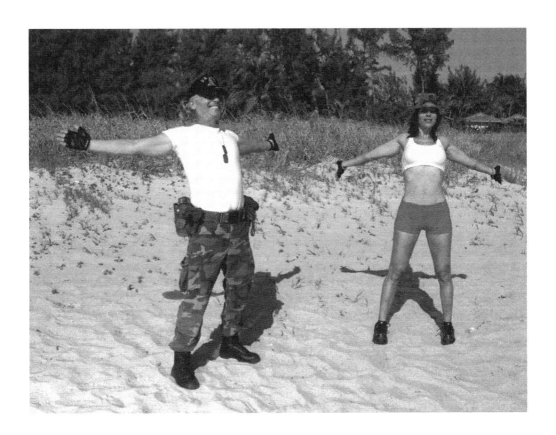

TRICEPS AND UPPER BACK

In the standing position with your feet shoulder-width apart, raise your right hand to the sky, then bend your elbow and place your right hand behind your back. Reach up over your head with your left hand and grab your right elbow. Now pull your right arm downward behind your back for a gentle stretch. Reverse arms and do it again. Hold for 15 to 20 seconds for each arm.

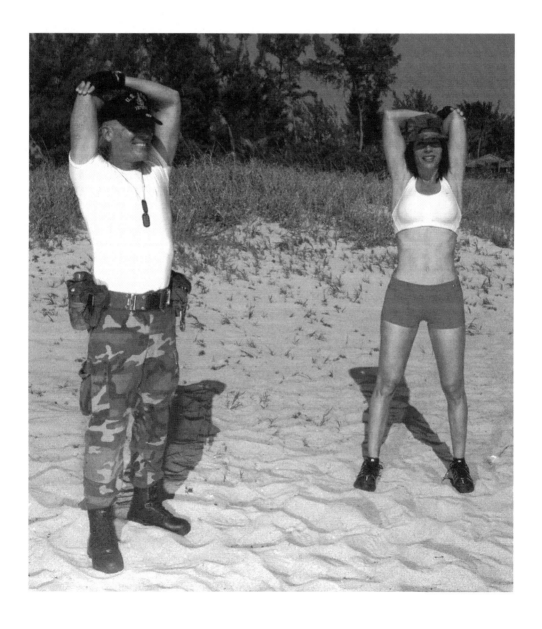

FOREARM STRETCH

After you've knocked out all those push-ups and pull-ups, you may experience some tightness in your forearms. This stretch will help to relieve the tightness. Reach your right arm out in front of you with your palm facing up as if you are making a hand signal for someone to stop. Reach over with your left hand and grab your right hand at the fingertips and gently pull back on your fingers. Hold for 15 to 20 seconds and then switch arms. For a variation, try this stretch with the fingers facing downward and then pull back with the other hand.

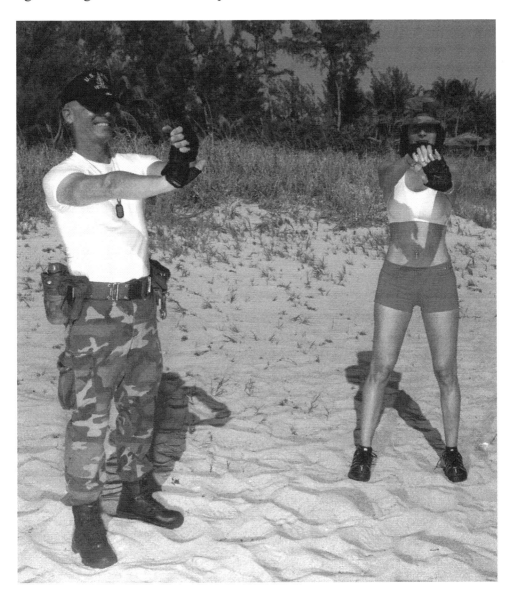

LOWER BACK STRETCH

You're flat on your back. Raise your head and pull your knees to yourstomach with your arms and hold for 15 to 20 seconds. This exercise is also called the cannonball if you happen to be jumping off a diving board.

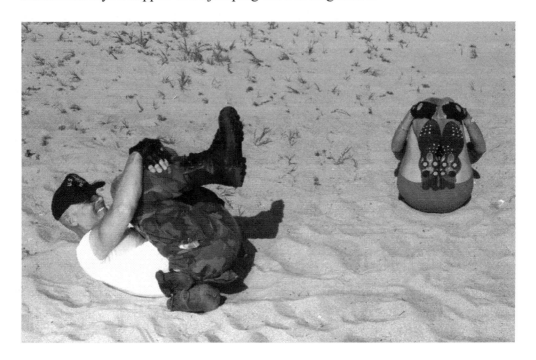

HIP ROTATIONS AS A FOUR-COUNT EXERCISE

This next stretch will be performed as a four-count exercise. Stand with your feet shoulder-width apart and your hands on your hips. You will count out loud and you will perform each movement using a slow and smooth motion, bending down as far as you can without hurting yourself. Here's the count: ONE, bow down forward and bring your upper body back to the upward position; TWO, now bend your upper body to the right and back to the starting position; THREE, bend your upper body backward and back to the starting position; FOUR, bend your upper body to the left and back to the starting position. For a warm-up stretch, you can perform one to five repetitions of this exercise.

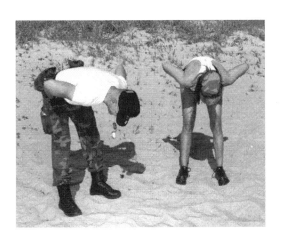
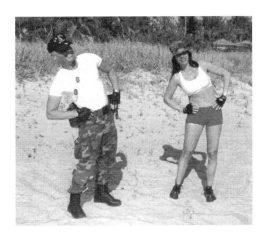

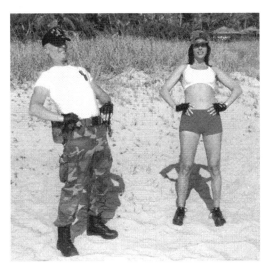
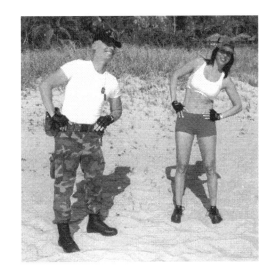

QUAD STRETCH

In the standing position, bend your right knee backward and grab your foot at the ankle with your right hand. Pull your foot to your butt while keeping your other leg straight and both legs close together. Hold for 15 to 20 seconds. Then switch sides and do the same. For support you can put the free hand against a tree, wall or on a rail.

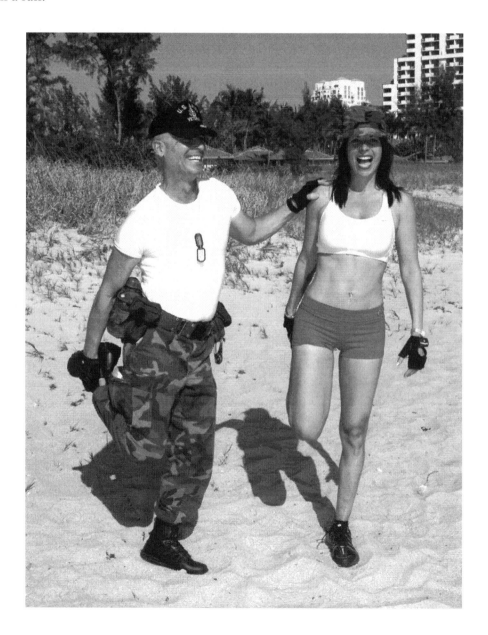

HAMSTRING STRETCH

In the standing position, extend your right leg forward and your left leg is back. Both legs are only about two feet apart, which means this is not a wide position for your legs. Now, while bending the left leg as a lever and your right leg is straight with knee locked, bend down towards your right leg and reach for the toes. You are stretching the hamstring of your right leg. To leverage that stretch, simply bend the left knee; the more you bend the left knee, the greater the stretch. No bouncing! Hold that stretch for 15 to 20 seconds. Switch positions of your legs and repeat the stretch.

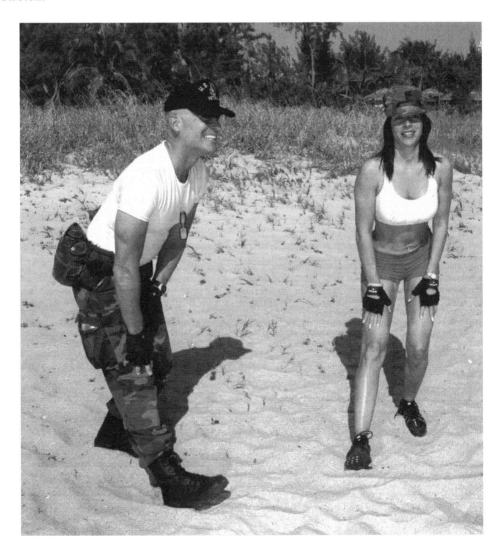

GROIN STRETCH (SEATED)

Sit on the ground with the bottoms of your feet together. Spread your legs with knees bent to have the bottoms of your feet touching. Place your hands around your feet and hold them together. Now bend forward and place your elbows on your knees and gently push downward with your elbows while keeping your head up. Hold for 15 to 20 seconds.

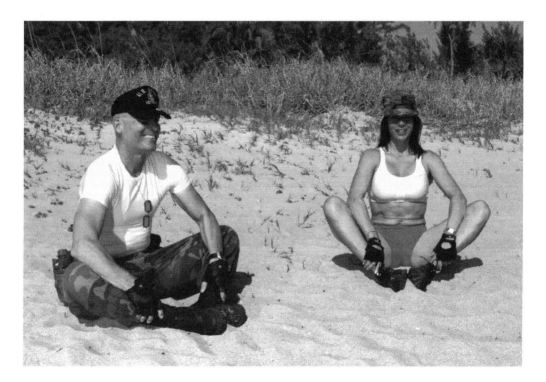

GROIN STRETCH (SEATED AND STRADDLED)

Sit on the ground with your legs straight and spread as far apart as you comfortably can without hurting yourself. Lean forward at your hips, keep your head up, and extend both arms and reach for your feet. Hold for about 15 to 20 seconds. To vary this stretch, turn to one side while trying to touch the toes. Hold for 15 to 20 seconds and then switch to the other side.

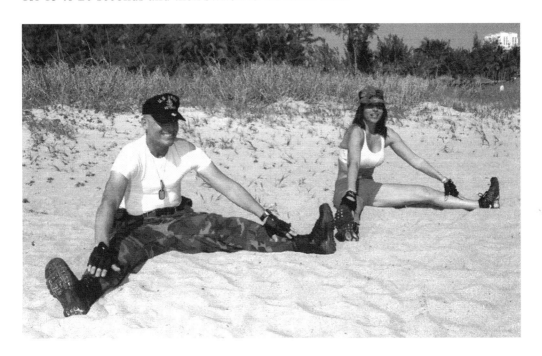

CHEST STRETCH, PARTNER ASSISTED

Sit with your back straight and raise your arms so that they are parallel to the ground and palms facing forward and elbows locked. Your partner stands behind you grasping the arms between the wrists and elbows. Your partner then gradually pulls both of your arms back until the stretch causes you mild discomfort. Hold the stretch for 15 to 20 seconds.

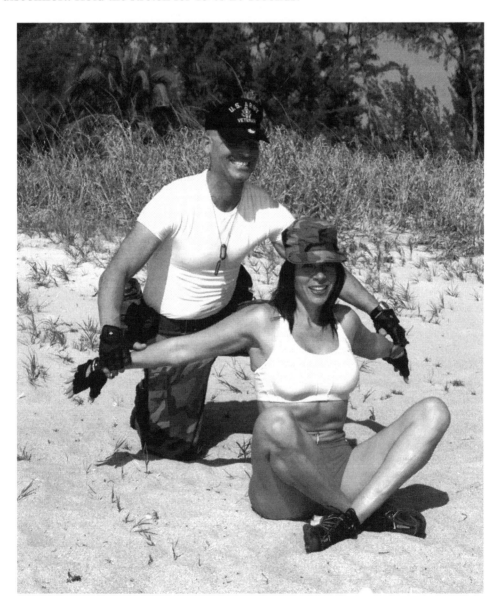

HAMSTRING, PARTNER ASSISTED

Sit straight up on the ground with your legs together and extended out, flat on the ground with knees locked. Your partner kneels down behind you. Your partner places light pressure on your upper back until you feel a mild discomfort. Hold for 15 to 20 seconds. Your partner can stand and push down on your back but be very careful! I once had a 300-pound guy in standing position push down on my back until my head was touching my legs and I'm not that flexible. It took me three months to completely recover. Light pressure and slight discomfort are words to be taken seriously when stretching. Remember, if you overextend connective tissue, it will tear.

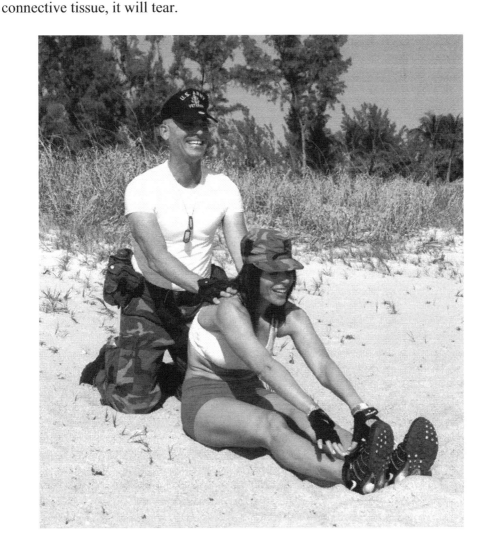

GROIN, PARTNER ASSISTED

Sit on the ground with your knees bent and the bottoms of your feet curved in together. Your partner kneels behind you and places light pressure on your knees with his hands and leans gently on your back with his chest until the stretch causes you mild discomfort. Hold this position for 15 to 20 seconds.

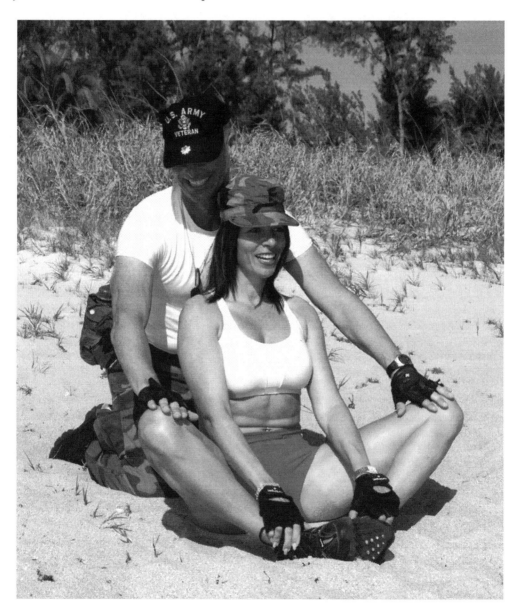

HAMSTRINGS AND GLUTS, PARTNER ASSISTED

Lie down on your back, raise your left leg and place your lower part of your left leg on your partner's right shoulder. You slowly stretch the hamstring and glutes by gradually bringing the straightened leg toward your head until you feel tension in the stretched muscles. Your partner then applies light pressure on your lower leg to help maintain or increase the stretch. You then isometrically contract your hamstrings and glutes for 5 to 10 seconds by attempting to move your leg downward and away from your head. Your partner steadily resists your efforts and does not allow any movement. Then, relax the hamstring and glute muscles. You then try to stretch them farther by using your partner's help and by contracting the hip flexor muscles (the illopsoas and quadriceps) and the tibialis anterior muscles for 5 to 10 seconds. Perform these stretches three times for each leg. Try to stretch a little farther each time.

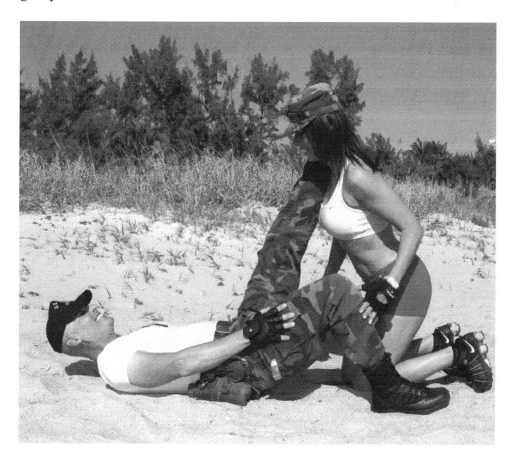

BICEPS AND CHEST

Using an object, such as a tree, pole or wall, place the palm of your right hand on the object with your arm extended and parallel to the ground. Now step forward with your right foot so that you gently stretch your biceps and chest muscles. Hold for 15 to 20 seconds. Switch sides and repeat.

Not the maker of plans and promises, but rather the one who offers faithful service in small matters. This is the person who is most likely to achieve what is good and lasting.

- Johann Wolfgang von Goethe

CALF STRETCH

Your left leg is forward and your right leg is as far back as you can bring it while maintaining the ball of your foot on the ground. Lean forward into your left leg and attempt to keep your right foot flat on the ground for a stretch of your right calf. Hold for 15 to 20 seconds. Switch and do the same with your left calf.

STANDING STRADDLE AND STRETCH

In the standing position, spread your legs as far as you comfortably can. Rotate your upper body (trunk) to the right and reach for the right foot by touching it or attempting to touch it. Hold for 10 to 20 seconds. Bring your trunk back up to the facing forward position while legs are still straddled and spread. This time rotate your trunk to the left and reach for the left foot. Hold for 10 to 20 seconds. Bring your trunk back up and face forward. Bend your trunk down to the middle while spreading your arms and reaching for each foot. Hold for 10 to 20 seconds.

ABS STRETCH

After completion of an abdominal exercise and while on your back in the prone position, briefly stretch your abs by raising your arms up over your head and parallel to the ground and legs extended. Hold for 10 seconds. Bend your knees and swivel your legs to the right. Hold for 10 seconds. Now swivel your knees to the left. Hold for 10 seconds. While your knees are bent, your arms are still up over your head to continue that abs stretch.

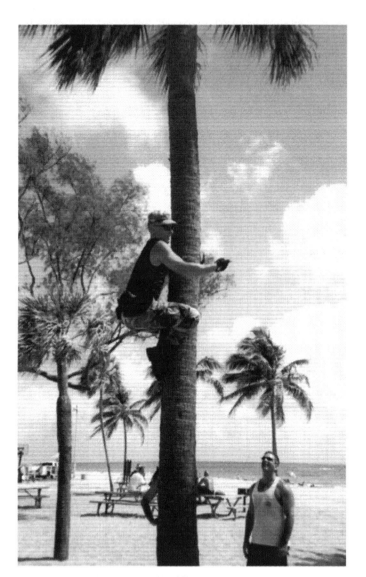

Col. Bob climbing Palm tree

Chapter Fourteen

Upper Body Without Weights

UPPER BODY WEIGHT EXERCISES

Upper body strength training without weights demonstrates the portability and flexibility of the human body when it comes to staying in shape. From a health standpoint, you do not need one single piece of equipment or some special place to stay lean and strong. Whether it's in your living room, bedroom, hotel room, on the patio, in the yard, the break room at work or in your office, you can immediately enjoy taking care of your strength training. The following exercises are all that you need. You will work the chest, arms, biceps, and triceps, upper and lower back.

REGULAR PUSH-UP

Let's move on to the best and most complete upper body exercise in the world. It's the push-up. All right, now get down with me for this one. Let's do it! Get down on all fours. Your feet are together, your body is straight. Your arms are a little more than shoulder-width apart and are spread in line with your chest. Go down to a 90 degree break in your elbows and come back up. Now, wasn't that easy? Yeah, I know. For a lot of you out there, it's pretty strenuous. That's OK. If you find you can only go down partially, you will still be working those muscles and you will get stronger and eventually be able go all the way down. I recommend to my clients to practice the regular push-up even though they cannot go all the way down and push their body back up. This approach is better than just performing knee push-ups.

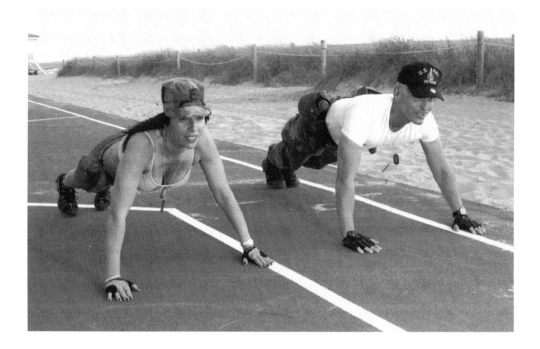

WIDE PUSH-UP

The wide (extra wide) push-up is performed the same way as the regular push-up with one exception. This time your hands are spread as wide as you can get them without collapsing. Your body is closer to the ground this time in the starting position. You will notice how the chest now enjoys a very beneficial workout along with your arms.

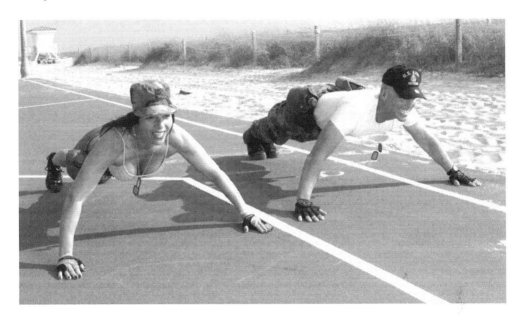

TRICEPS PUSH-UP

Now get down for another great variation of the push-up. This time your hands are close together and your feet are spread about shoulder width for stability. Go down to the point where your chest is almost touching the ground and come back up. Feel those triceps work? You'll notice that this one feels more strenuous than the regular push-up.

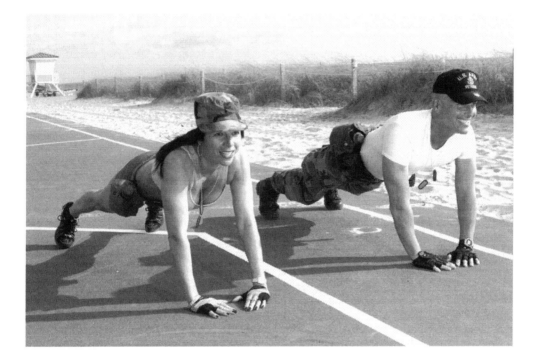

FOUR COUNT PUSH-UP

Now let's put some real excitement into the push-up. These are regular push-ups with a twist. This time you will stop and pause between each motion. You will notice that you will get even more benefit from this strength training exercise. It's a four count. Here we go and ONE, lower your body (pause); TWO, raise it back up (pause); THREE, lower your body (pause); FOUR, raise it back up (pause). That's one repetition. Try five to ten reps and count them out loud. The count is one, two, three, ONE; one, two, three, TWO; one, two, three, THREE; and so on.

KNEE PUSH-UPS, 45 DEGREES

Get down on your knees for this push-up which simply means that you will be pumping less body weight. Your legs are at a 45 degree angle. You can actually perform all of the previously mentioned push-ups using this position.

KNEE PUSH-UPS, 90 DEGREES

This push-up position will allow you to lessen the body weight even more than the 45 degree angle push-up. The various types of push-ups described previously can be performed using the 90 degree push-up.

REGULAR PULL-UP

The pull-up is an advanced upper body exercise. The bar should be above your head to start when in the standing position. Reach up and grab the bar with palms facing away and hands just a little more than shoulder width apart. Keep your body stable by bending your knees back and crossing your legs. Avoid any rocking motion. Now pull the body up to where the chin is just above the bar and back down in the arms extended position. That's one pull-up.

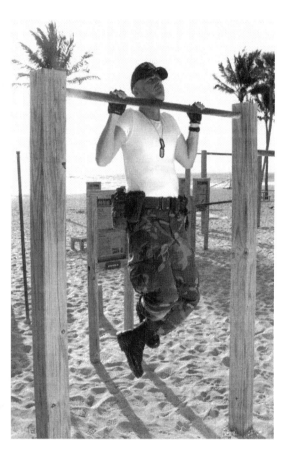
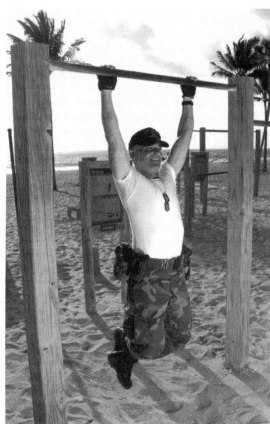

REVERSE PULL-UP

Facing the bar, reach up and grab it with your palms facing toward you and hands about shoulder width apart and arms completely extended. Pull your body up to the point where your chin is just above the bar and then back down to the starting position. Use a smooth motion in both directions and not too fast for any of the pull-ups. Concentrate on form and avoid the use of momentum so that you continually work those muscles.

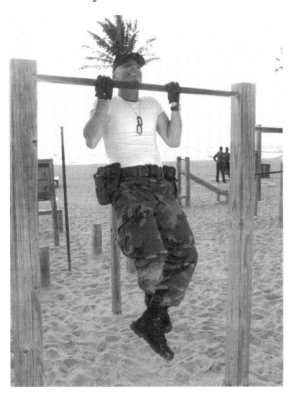
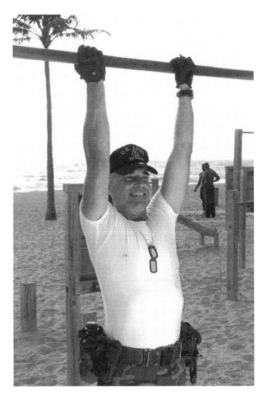

TRICEPS PULL-UP

Facing the bar, reach up and grab it with your palms facing away from you and hands completely together with thumbs touching. Keep your body stable by bending your knees back and crossing your legs. Avoid any rocking motion to concentrate on form. Now pull the body up to where the chin is just above the bar and back down in the arms extended position.

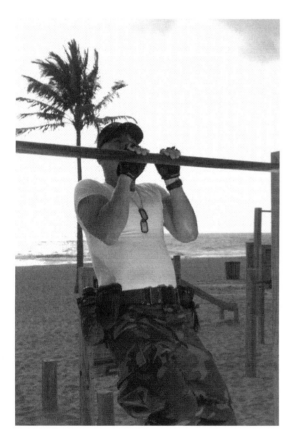
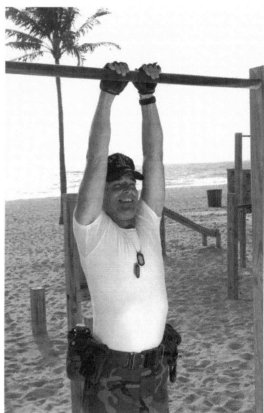

EXTRA WIDE PULL-UP

Facing the bar, reach up and grab it with your palms facing away from you and hands as wide as you can go. Keep your body stable by bending your knees back and crossing your legs. Avoid any rocking motion to concentrate on form. Now pull the body up to where the chin is just above the bar and back down in the arms extended position.

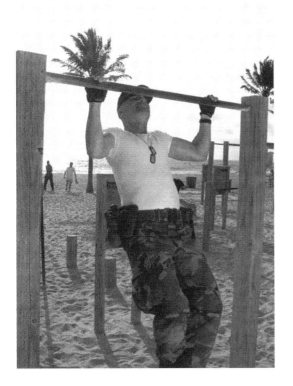 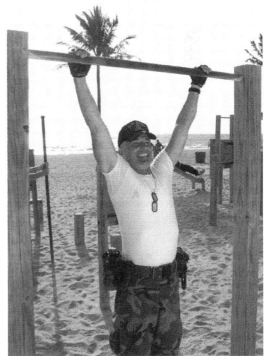

CLIFFHANGERS

Now I know very few of you will ever be in a situation where you're hanging over a cliff. Nevertheless, a little cliffhanging strength never hurt and it's awesome for strengthening the arms and back. Face the bar and then step under it and turn facing left. Reach up and grab the bar with hands staggered. Grab the bar with your left hand on the left side of the bar and with your right hand on the right side. Your right hand is just in front of your left hand. Pull your body up on the right side and touch your shoulder to the bar, then lower your body while keeping your legs off of the ground. Do it again with the left side. Count each side as one rep and perform reps in even numbers.

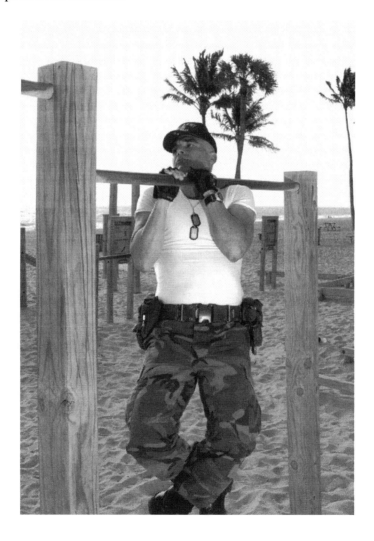

ASSISTED PULL-UPS

Any of the variation of pull-ups can be performed with a partner who either grabs your feet or grabs you around the waist to assist you. No tickling permitted unless you want an additional challenge!

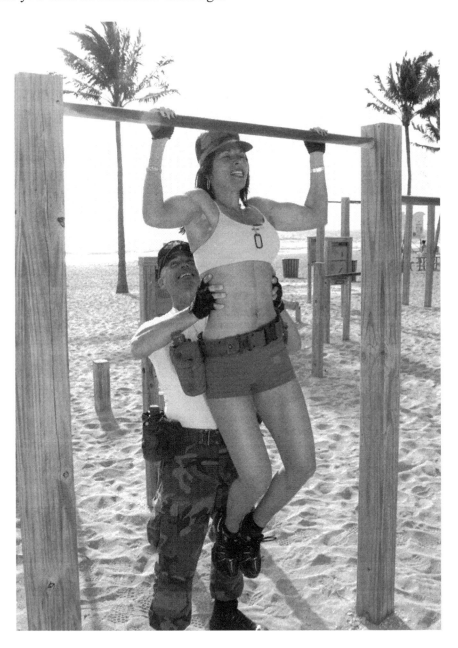

STRAIGHT LEG INCLINES (USING THE LOW BAR FOR PULL-UPS)

Using the low bar that is about three feet off the ground, get under the bar and grab it with hands a little more than shoulder width apart. All types of the above pull-ups can be done in this position. Your body is straight and arms extended in the starting position. Pull your body up until your chest is close to the bar and then back down. That's one repetition.

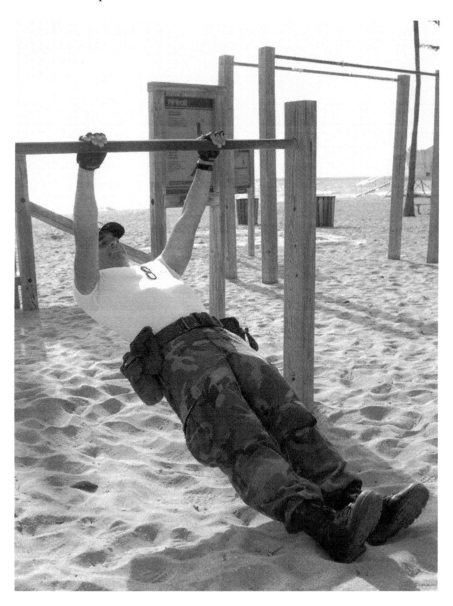

REGULAR DIPS

I know you ladies are always especially interested in working the triceps to look really good in that sleeveless dress. I've got a solution. It's called the dip. You will need a sturdy object like a chair or bench or rail that is anywhere from one to three feet off of the ground. Have a seat on the bench or chair and place your hands on each side of your body as close as you can with your fingers facing forward and curled over the edge of the bench. Your legs are about shoulder width apart with a greater than ninety degree bend. Raise your rearward anatomy off of the bench and lower your body while keeping your back close to the bench, both while going down and coming back up.

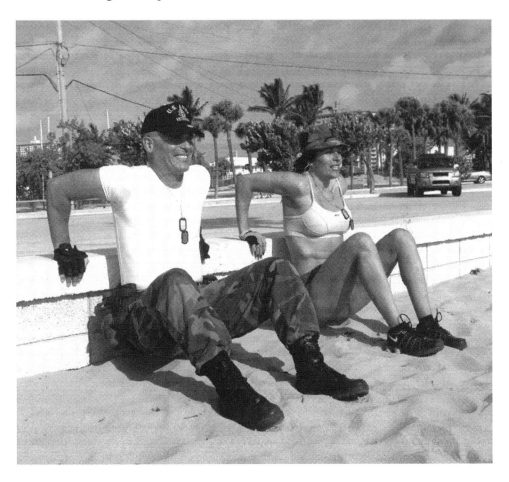

STRAIGHT LEG DIPS

Get in the same position as with the regular dips. This time, raise your right leg with knee locked and parallel to the ground. Knock out five reps just for fun. Notice the difference compared with the regular dips? Switch and raise the left leg this time. This gets me excited just writing about it! I know how good it feels!

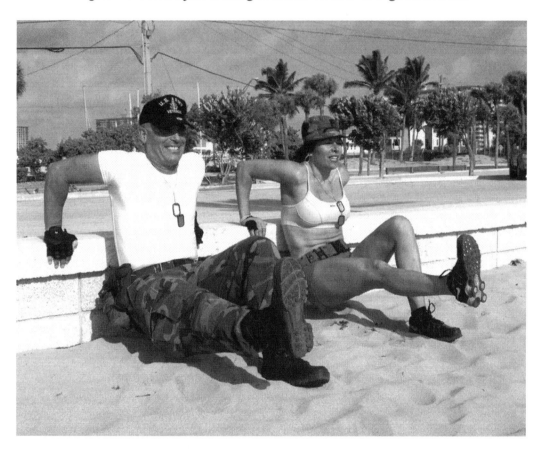

Upper Body Workout and Reps Guide

Exercises	Beginner	Intermediate	Advanced
Regular Push-up	2 - 20	20 - 30	30 - 100
Wide Push-up	2 - 15	15 - 25	25 - 60
Tricep Push-up	2 - 8	8 - 20	20 - 50
4-count Push-up	2 - 5	8 - 20	20 - 40
Knee Push-ups, 45 Degrees	10 - 20	20 - 60	60 - 100
Knee Push-ups, 90 Degrees	10 - 20	20 - 60	60 - 100
Regular Pull-up	0 - 5	5 - 10	10 - 25
Reverse Pull-up	0 - 5	5 - 15	15 - 30
Hands-together Tricep Pull-up	0 - 3	3 - 10	10 - 20
Extra Wide Pull-up	0 - 2	2 - 5	5 - 15
Cliffhangers	0 - 2	2 - 10	10 - 20
Assisted Pull-ups	3 - 10	10 - 30	30 - 40
Straight Leg Inclines	2 - 8	8 - 20	20 - 40
Regular Dips	5 - 15	15 -40	40 - 100
Straight Leg Dips, each leg	5 - 10	10 - 20	20 - 40

Never measure the height of a mountain until you have reached the top. Then you will see how low it was.

- Dag Hammarskjold

Chapter Fifteen

Upper Body
With Resistance Bands

Resistance Band
Strength Training

I want to introduce you to the most portable and affordable piece of equipment you can use for your workouts anywhere, anytime. It's called the resistance band or tube. It is an oversized rubber band with handles on each end for your hands. There are many manufacturers out there. I prefer the bands by the company, SPRI which you can find at my website TheHealthColonel.com. There are six levels of resistance, all color coded:

WHICH RESISTANCE BAND/TUBE IS RIGHT FOR YOU?

You need to go by your *current* strength and fitness level, not by what you would *like* to be in order to work your muscles effectively and to prevent injuries.

Lavender - **very light** - rehab, medical conditions and frail people.
Yellow - **light** - children, rehab, some women and seniors, 2-5 lbs.
Green - **medium** - average (inactive) women and some older men, 5-10 lbs.
Red - **heavy** - average men and active, fairly strong women, 11-16 lbs.
Blue - **extra-heavy** - active men and very strong women, 17-22 lbs.
Purple/black - **ultra-heavy** - strong men or women bodybuilders, 23-30 lbs.

Choosing a band will depend upon the type of workout you are doing. If you are performing high reps of 50 to 100 you will probably use at least one level down compared to performing just 10 to 20 reps per set. Your fatigue level while performing circuit training (combined cardio and strength training) will also play a roll when choosing a resistance band. You may or may not choose a high resistance level depending upon how intense you conduct your circuit training.

Let's move on to the various upper body exercises with the resistance band.

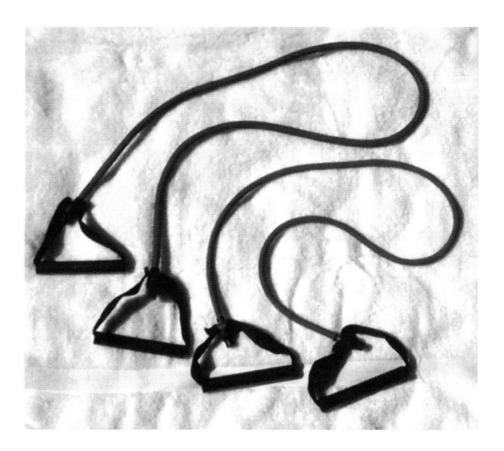

BICEP CURLS

Grab each handle with your left and right hand. Your feet are shoulder width apart and you are standing firmly on the band with the band in the center of your shoes. Bend your knees slightly to stabilize your lower back with your palms facing out and your arms extended down. Pull the band up to your shoulder joint and resist it going down.

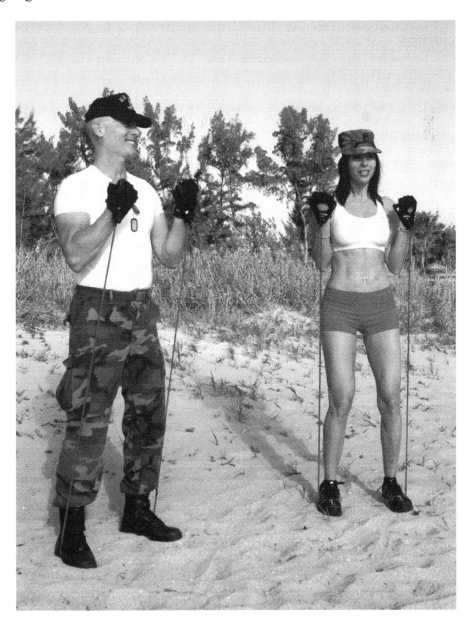

UPRIGHT ROW

Grab each handle with your left and right hand. Two feet on the band, your feet are shoulder width apart with a slight bend in the knees to stabilize your lower back. With both wrists hanging down, pull the band up to your shoulder joint while maintaining your wrists in the down position and then back to the starting position while resisting it going down. Let's practice. And one, two, three, four, five.

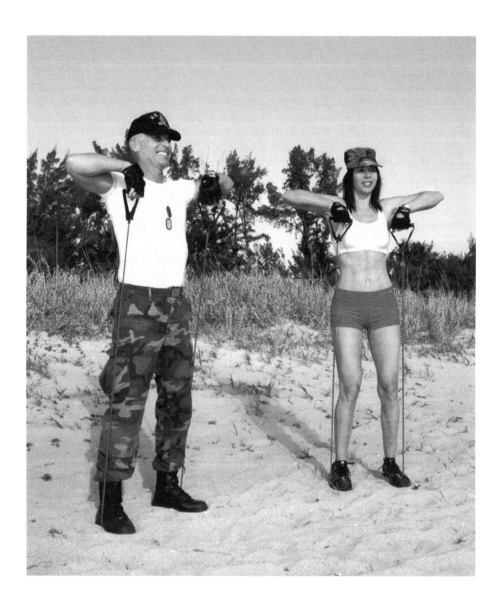

SHOULDER PRESS

Grab each handle with your left and right hand. Your left foot is on the band in the center of the shoe. Step through the band/tube with your right foot. Bring your arms up to a ninety degree break in your elbows. Your wrists are straight and the band is behind the arms.

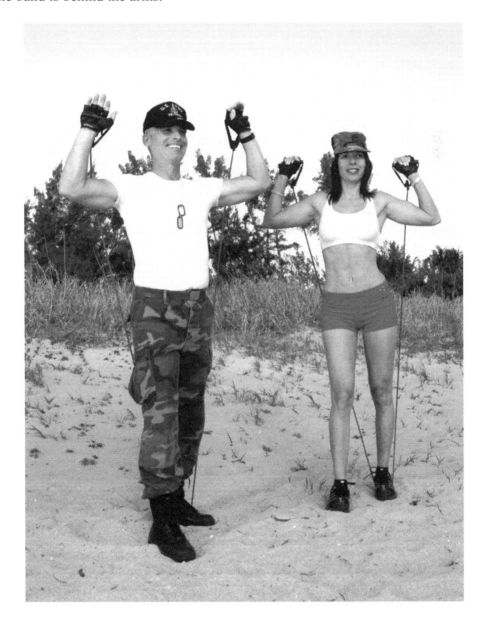

FRONT RAISE

Grab each handle with your left and right hand. This one's a little more strenuous. Your left foot is forward and on the band. Extend your arms forward, lock your elbows and hold your wrists straight with palms facing down. Pull the band upward to where the arms are parallel to the ground and resist it going back down.

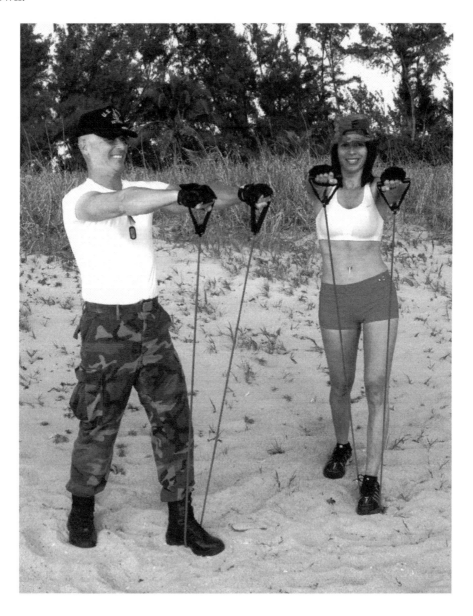

SIDE LATERAL RAISE

Grab each handle with your left and right hand. This one is similar to the front raise, except that the arms are extended and raised at the sides. Your left foot is forward and on the band. Extend your arms out to the sides, lock your elbows with arms straight and hold your wrists straight with your palms facing down. Pull the band up until the arms are parallel to the ground and resist it going back down.

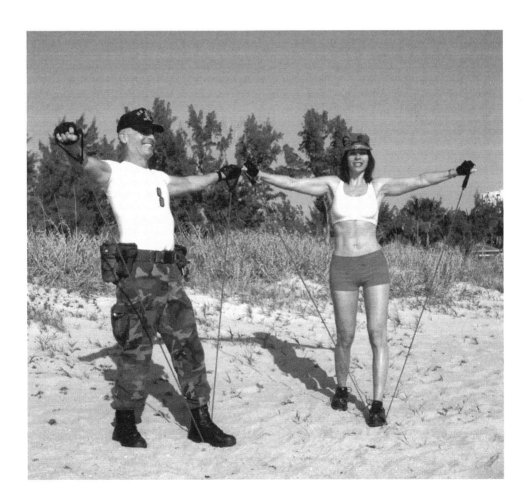

STANDING ROW

Grab each handle with your left and right hand. This next exercise will really demonstrate the versatility of the resistance band and how to incorporate your environment into the workout. Wrap the band around a tree or pole. We're going to perform a standing row exercise. Your band is wrapped around the tree. Get some resistance in the band with palms facing inward and an exaggerated bend in your knees to stabilize your lower back. Your back is straight and arms completely extended for the starting position. Pull back on the band in line with your chest and resist it going all the way back out. Find a distance that will allow you to have enough resistance to work your muscles and still perform the complete range of motion. That's one rep.

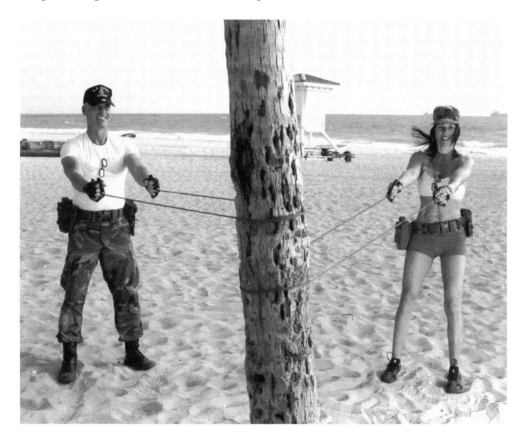

STANDING TRICEPS PUSH

Grab each handle with your left and right hand. Let's move on to another great triceps exercise with the resistance band. It's called the standing triceps push. Take the band in your right hand and place the other end on the ground in front of your right foot. Place your right foot six to eight inches into the band and firmly onto to the band with the ball of your foot so that it doesn't slip. Now step forward with your left foot, while keeping your right foot on the band. Take your right hand with the band and bring it up behind your head. The starting position is with the hand lowered behind your head. Push up on the band until the arm is completely extended. That's one rep. Switch hands and feet and do the same thing with the left side of your body.

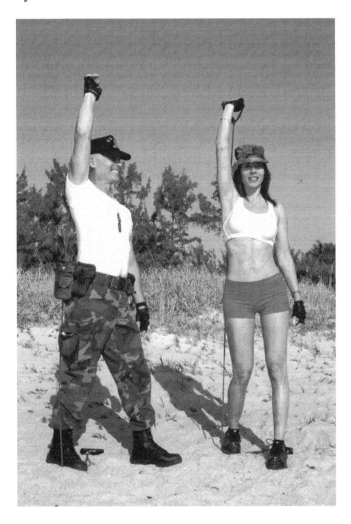

REVERSE CURLS

Grab each handle with your left and right hand. Here's a great way to work the forearms. Reverse curls. Your feet are shoulder width apart and standing firmly on the band with the band in the center of your shoe, maintain a slight bend in your knees to stabilize the lower back. Your palms are facing back and your arms are extended down. Pull the band up to your shoulder joint and resist it going down. This will feel awkward and unusual at first.

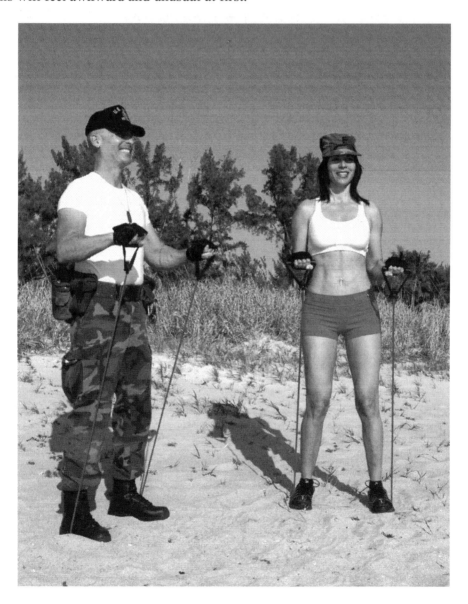

PARTNER ASSISTED STANDING ARM CURL

Both you and your partner can perform this exercise together. You and your partner face each other. Two resistance bands of the same resistance level are used for this exercise. Each person grabs one handle of the same resistance band with the right hand and one handle of the other _____ resistance band with the left. Now step back from each other to increase tension and stand with feet shoulder width apart and slight bend in the knees. Your arms are fully extended with palms facing up in the starting position. To execute this exercise you and your partner curl your arms upward while keeping your body stationary. You are not lifting your arms. You are merely curling upward and bending at the elbow and then back to the extended position. That's one repetition.

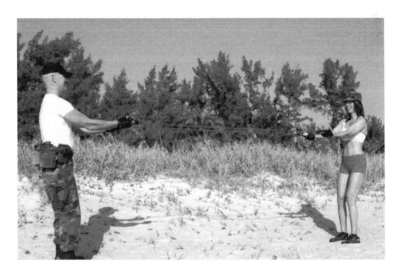

Resistance Band Upper Body Workout Reps Guide			
Exercises	**Beginner**	**Intermediate**	**Advanced**
Bicep Curls	5 - 30	30 - 60	60 - 100
Upright Row	5 - 40	40 - 60	60 - 100
Shoulder Press	3 - 10	10 - 15	15 - 40
Front Raise	5 - 10	10 - 15	15 - 20
Side Lateral Raise	5 - 10	10 - 15	15 - 20
Standing Row	10 - 40	40 - 70	70 - 100
Standing Triceps Push	5 - 10	10 - 20	20 - 30
Reverse Curls	4 - 15	15 - 20	20 - 40
Partner Assisted Standing Arm Curl	10 - 20	20 - 30	30 - 60

STANDING ROW WITH THE THERA-BAND LATEX RESISTIVE EXERCISE BAND

As with the standing row using the resistance tube wrapped around the tree the theraband offers the same kind of flexibility and portability. This type of band has no handles so you wrap each end around your hands and hold tightly.

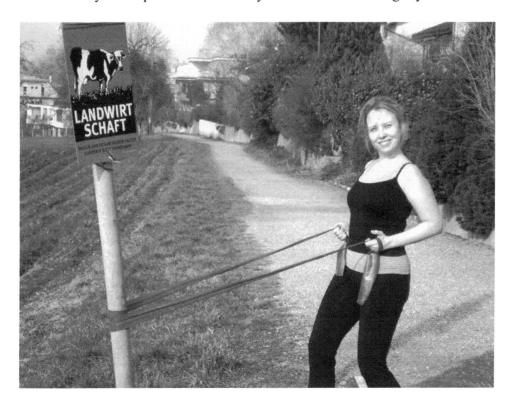

Prone Position Exercises With The Thera-Band

The sky is truly the limit with these exercises. Have you ever seen such a smile?

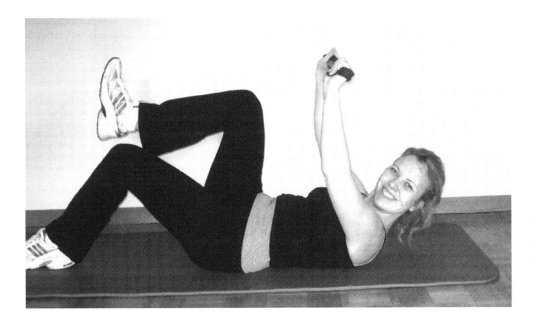

There are no hopeless situations, there are only people who have grown hopeless about them.

- Clare Boothe Luce

Chapter Sixteen

Lower Body Without Weights

LOWER BODY STRENGTH TRAINING

BODY PARTS WORKED: HIPS, THIGHS, BUTT, QUADS AND HAMSTRINGS

The strength training exercises described in this chapter will equip you to work your lower body completely independent of exercise equipment. For the busy person, these exercises are optimal. Many of these can even be performed within the constrains of a work cubicle. Imagine calling a brief time out in your cubicle "jungle" with all heads popping up and then performing a squat or some other exercise together. This may very well be as entertaining as Meerkat Manor on Animal Planet. Add some music and MTV will be calling. What a way to combine team building, having fun and it will certainly loosen up the atmosphere and reduce stress. By getting that blood flowing from all that sedentary work, it'll even promote increased performance.

SQUATS

Your feet are shoulder width apart with your arms on your hips or hands together with elbows bent and your head up and upper body in a natural upright position – not the bending over forward ski position. Bend your knees to a 90 degree break making sure that your knee does not go past your big toe. Then bring your body back up to the upright position. That's one repetition.

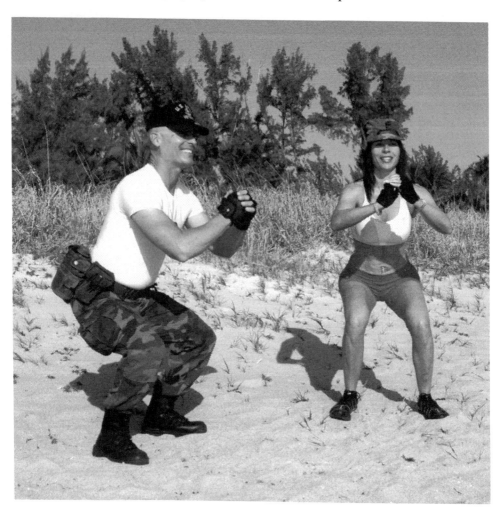

WALKING LUNGES

Pretend you are carrying two full buckets of water to emphasize good posture of your upper body in the upright position. What I want you to do is step forward with your right foot to the point where your knees are bent at 90 degrees. Your knee of the forward leg should not go past your big toe. Pause briefly and then step all the way through with your left leg. Pause briefly. Now continue this exercise. As a matter of fact, why not just go for a walk like this? Who knows? You may strike up some interesting conversation along the way.

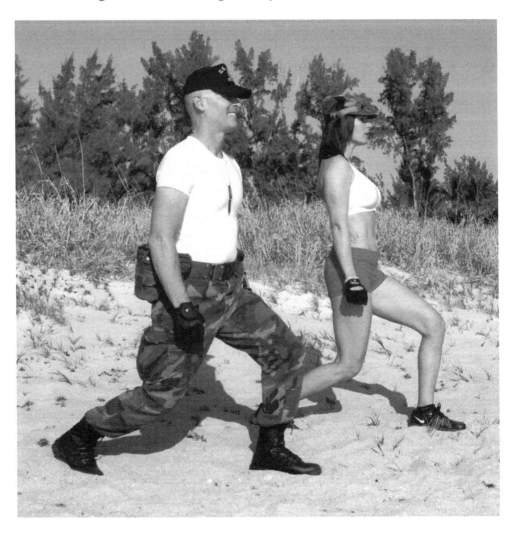

STATIONERY LUNGES

As with the walking lunge, pretend you are carrying two full buckets of water. Step forward with your right foot to the point where your knees are bent at 90 degrees. Your knee of the forward leg should not go past your big toe. Now simply lower your body to the point where your knees are bent at 90 degrees. Then bring your body back up. That's one repetition. For example, do twenty reps in this position and then switch off with the left leg forward and do twenty more.

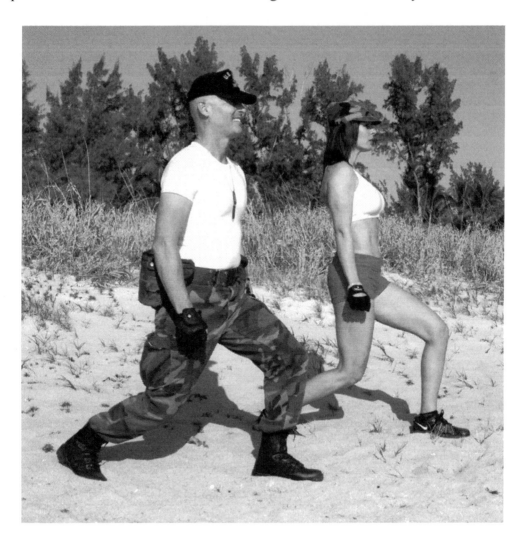

DIRTY DOGS

Get down on all fours with your head facing forward. You will need your visualization skills for this. Imagine it's time to take Fido around the block for those customary stops along the way. You now move up to the first tree and Fido stops and raises his leg smartly to take care of business. This is a great opportunity to mark your territory. When taking on any project or task in life, it's essential that you take ownership (= mark your territory). Now raise your right leg with the knee bent just like Fido and lower it again. That's one rep. For example, do twenty reps with the right leg and switch off and do twenty with the left. Now here's a test question for you. Why do you want to perform the same number of reps for both legs? Hint: How would a lopsided butt look? Spare me the thought!

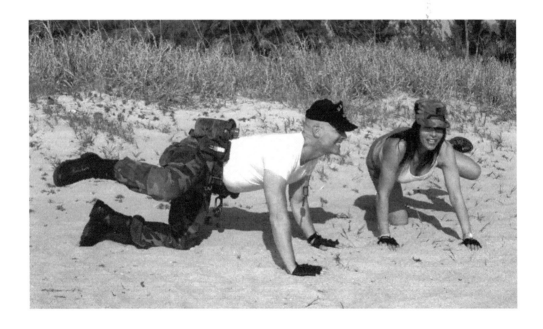

LEG THRUSTS

Get down on all fours facing forward. Take your right leg and thrust itstraight back while holding it parallel to the ground with the toes pointed downward, then thrust the leg back to the position where you attempt to touch your chest with your knee. That is one rep. Count the rep with the straight leg position. Switch legs to work the other side. For example, do twenty reps with the right leg, then do twenty with the left. As with many of those body weightexercises there are many variations that can be performed. This is just one of them.

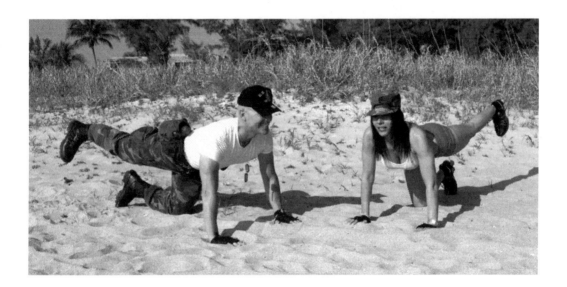

STANDING CRUNCHES

Stand upright with your left leg forward and your right leg back. Now thrust the right knee up to the point where you attempt to touch your chest with your knee and back down to the starting position. Switch legs and work the other side. Contract your abs while thrusting your knee to your chest.

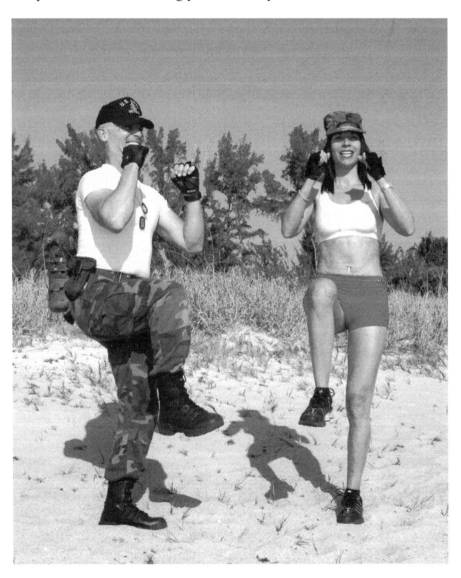

ALTERNATING SIDE LEG RAISES (4-COUNT EXERCISE)

Stand with feet shoulder width apart and with bent elbows and hands together just about chest high. Now squat down to the point where your legs are at a 90 degree angle. Make sure your knee does not go past your big toe. Here's the 4-count: ONE, squat to 90 degrees; TWO, lift (not kick) your left leg out to about hip height to the extended position with knees locked; THREE, back to the squat position; FOUR, lift (not kick) your right leg to about hip height while keeping it straight. That is one rep. 10 reps are a good number per set.

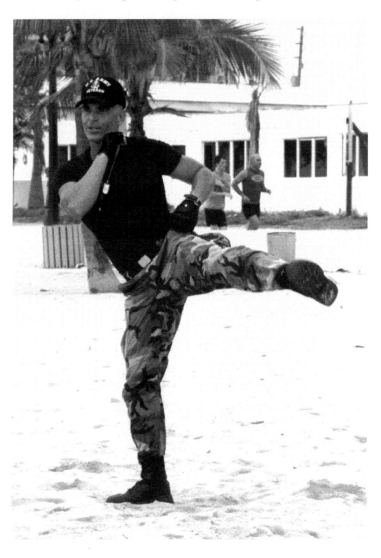

Lower Body Workout Reps Guide			
Exercises	**Beginner**	**Intermediate**	**Advanced**
Squats	20 - 40	40 - 100	100 - 200
Standing Lunges, each leg	5 - 20	20 - 60	60 - 100
Dirty Dogs, each leg	5 - 10	10 - 40	40 - 80
Leg Thrusts, each leg	5 - 20	20 - 50	50 - 80
Standing Crunches, each leg	10 - 30	30 - 60	60 - 100
Alternating Side Leg Raise (Lift)	10 - 15	15 - 30	30 - 70

To be yourself in a world that is constantly trying to make you something else is the greatest accomplishment.

- Ralph Waldo Emerson

Chapter Seventeen

Jump, Kick and Punch

BODY PARTS WORKED

HEART, LUNGS, BUTT, HIPS, THIGHS, CALVES, QUADS, HAMSTRINGS, ARMS

The number and variations of body weight exercises are limitless. The following exercises are not included in the upper and lower body weight exercises because I consider them to be in a category of their own. This does not mean that you won't be working the upper or lower body. The opposite is true. Remember, our bodies are designed to work in sync. These basic supplemental exercises add to your arsenal of body weight exercises which is what you need to keep your program interesting, fun and health focused.

JUMPING JACKS

A callisthenic workout is never complete without jumping jacks. Stand with feet together and arms at your sides. You're going to need a little bounce for this one. Jump to the spread leg position and land your feet back on the ground while you bring your arms together over your head (arms are raised and extended over your head). Then immediately jump back to the starting position with feet together while bringing your arms back down to your sides. This is a smooth motion. Jump out. Then jump back to the starting position. That is one repetition. Perform 50 to 100 reps. Of course you can start out with less, if you feel the need. This is a high impact exercise. If you have any medical issues with your knees or ankles, please consult your physician. Try modifying the exercise by spreading your legs partially and not jumping as high if you have a medical issue that allows you to modify the exercise.

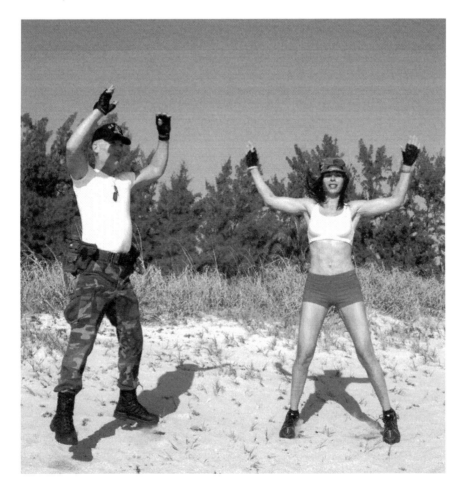

WIND MILLS

Stand with your feet wider than shoulder width apart and arms extended parallel to the ground, out to your sides and palms facing down with elbowslocked. Bend over and take your right hand diagonally across your body andreach for your left foot while extending your left arm pointing towards the sky and then back to the starting position with both arms extend out and parallel to the ground. In the starting position you're not bent over but standing erect between each repetition. Perform 10 to 20 reps.

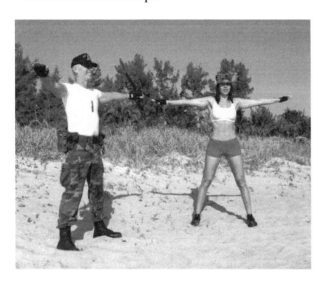

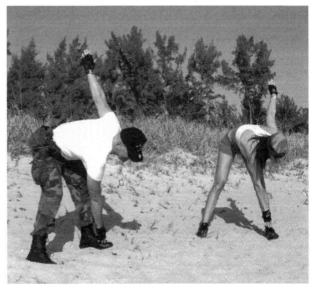

KICK

Your right leg is back. Your left leg is forward. Perform a snap kick with the right leg by thrusting it out and kicking about kneecap high and then back to the starting position. That is one repetition. Switch legs to work the other side. For example, if you are performing thirty reps, work first one leg with all thirty and then the other. Count the reps with the leg in the extended (kick) position. Perform 30 to 60 reps with each leg.

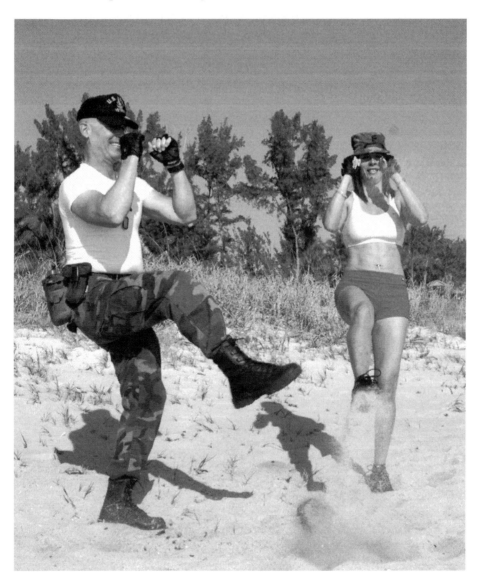

SIDE PUNCH

Your legs are shoulder width apart and fists are clenched and positioned in front of your face. Now punch your right fist to the left and snap it back to the starting position. Then punch your left fist to the right and snap it back to the starting position. Note that you are swiveling your hips for each punch and looking in the direction of your punch. This is a four count exercise. ONE; your right arm punches out to the left; TWO, your right arm is back to the starting position; THREE, your left arm punches out to the right; FOUR, your left arm is back to the starting position. That is one repetition. Perform 40 to 80 reps per set.

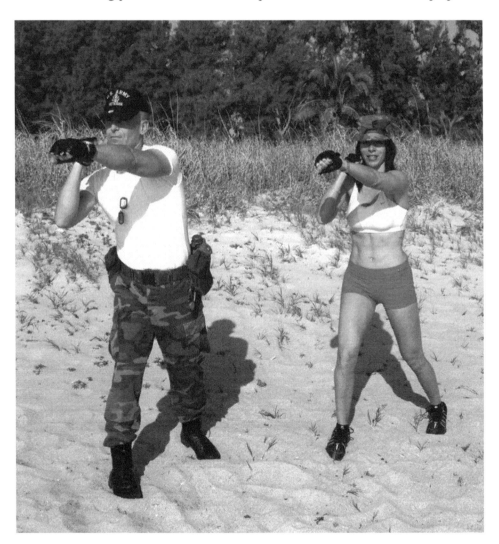

TOE RAISERS

Your feet are shoulder width apart with arms raised as if you are under arrest. Now reach down and touch your stomach, then your toes, then your stomach and back up to the starting position. This is a four count exercise. ONE, touch your stomach; TWO, touch your toes; THREE, touch your stomach; FOUR, back to the starting position with both arms raised above your head and extended. That is one
repetition. Perform 50 to 100 reps. Some of you are asking, "Why toe raisers?" Well, you can add a calf raise to this exercise by taking it up on your toes when you reach for the sky. Now you know why they're called toe raisers.

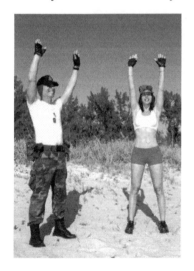
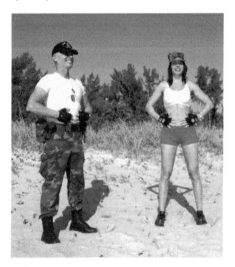

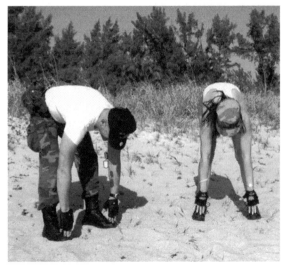

Chapter Eighteen

Cardio and Agility Drills

BODY PARTS WORKED

LUNGS, HEART, HIPS, THIGHS, CALVES, BUTT, ABS AND LOWER BACK

It's time to add some fun and games to your workout with some cardio and agility drills. Always consider your physical activity a dynamic and not static process. Make it a game. Think variety. Incorporate your environment into your workout. Though these drills call for the use of cones, you could use stones are even trees and bushes or chairs to run around. Always keep safety in mind.

BACKPEDAL/SPRINT DRILL (STAGGERED CONES)

Six cones will be needed for this drill. Place one cone as the starting point and the other five are placed like spokes in a wheel at different lengths (10 to 20 yards) from the starting cone and each of them about five yards apart. Each of the five cones will be placed at the 10, 12, 1 and 2 o'clock positions. Sprint to the 10 o'clock cone and backpedal back to the starting cone. Do this with each cone in the "spoke" until all are completed.

ZIGZAG SPRINT DRILL WITH CONES

Using six cones, stagger them in such a way that you will have to zigzag around each of them in order. This is a sprinting drill. Each cone should be about 5 yards apart. You will sprint around each cone until you have zigzagged through all the cones and then back again. The cones will be placed in two rows.

BOX DRILL WITH CONES

Using four cones form a box on your lawn. The cones can be about 25 yards apart although you my vary that distance as you like. You are standing at the first cone. You will sprint to the second cone. You will perform a lateral or sideways move to the third cone. You will back pedal to the fourth cone. You will sprint back to the first cone. Please note that you can simply just sprint to each cone or you can mix and match your own moves between each of the cones.

SUICIDES

This is a simple drill with a high cardio impact. Place one cone as the starting point and the other cone anywhere from 20 to 50 yards out. Sprint out and back, out and back, out and back, and so forth. I think you get the point. You can simply make this one a timed event with everyone at their own pace. When performing this as a group the great benefit is that no one really ever falls behind. As a matter of fact, you really can't tell who's ahead and who's behind. Regardless of fitness level all team members will enjoy a great cardio blast with this drill. I'm sure you'll notice the fatigue very quickly on this one.

FORWARD-BACK-LEFT-RIGHT

This can be done in a group with a group leader guide or by yourself. The guide leader will call the signals randomly to change direction. Don't run into any trees or fall in a ditch going backwards! The commands are simple: FORWARD, BACK, LEFT, RIGHT. The commands FORWARD and BACK simply mean to run forward and backward. The commands LEFT and RIGHT mean run sideways to the left and to the right. This is lots of fun and a great way to work on the agility and the lower body. How long? As long as the guide leader is yelling out commands. The leader can either face the group and give hand signals as well or he or she can join in with the group and shout out the commands.

RUN FORREST RUN!

I'm sure most of you have seen the movie "Forrest Gump." Once Forrest started running, he didn't know when to stop. For most of us out there, it's more like not knowing when to start. I had to specifically mention running. What I mean is anything that leaves the realm of simply walking. Keep in mind that running (jogging) is a great way to work the heart, lungs, butt, hips, thighs, quads, hamstrings and much more.

LEARN TO THROTTLE YOUR RUNNING PACE

Before ever stopping, try throttling it down to a slower running or jogging pace first. This works on two things: your mental strength and it keeps you on the run. Unless you are sprinting, your upper body should be relaxed and only your legs and lungs should be working. No feet dragging or pavement pounding is permitted unless you have a sudden urge to hear me say, "Drop and give me twenty!" Foot dragging or scraping or foot pounding is a recipe for injuries to connective tissue in your lower body. Your stride and your body mechanics should be smooth. You land on your heels and roll across your foot. You're not really going to be thinking about this when you run. Just check yourself every now and then for smooth, efficient running mechanics.

Your breathing – as with all exercises - should be natural and should not be heard, and the mouth should not be making some unnatural forms that you've seen in some of those workout videos or in the gym. You're getting some of the Health Colonel's philosophy about breathing.

YOUR BODY IS DESIGNED TO RUN

Oh, and by the way, your body was designed to run, contrary to some of the things you may have heard. The latest research has determined the gluts – that's that rearward anatomy, also known as the butt – are not really working when walking. I want to emphasize the running because it is also working the complete lower body to include the lower back and abs. (Source: NewScientist.com: July 30, 2007 "Duplicate genes help humans go the extra mile," by Roxanne Khamsi; Discovermagazine.com, May 28, 2006, "Born To Run, Biomechanical research reveals a surprising key to the survival of our species: Humans are built to outrun nearly every other animal on the planet over long distances." by Ingfei Chen)

Run Forrest run!			
	Beginner	**Intermediate**	**Advanced**
Run 1 Mile	11:00 - 18:00	8:00 - 11:00	5:00 - 8:00
Run 2 Miles	16:00 - 30:00	14:00 - 16:00	10:00 - 14:00

BACKPEDAL

Who says you always have to run or walk forward? There are actually backward track races. Now, I do have to admit that the falls during these races are quite spectacular and a sight to see. Ouch! Backpedaling is a great way to recruit those lower body muscles in a different way. Just make sure that you use your peripheral vision so that you don't run into that tree or signpost and definitely do not run backwards (or forwards) in traffic. I provided some great entertainment during a group class on the beach when I ran right into a palm tree. Don't worry. No injuries except for my pride.

TUG-O-WAR

Remember those days in school or summer camp when you would engage in a tug-o-war competition with a rope? Well, this happens to be an exercise (or game) that you can't do alone. You'll need a rope of special tug-o-war material with loops. Do an internet search and you will find lots of options.

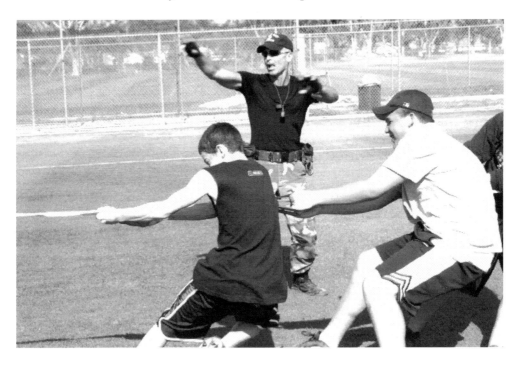

Run, Jump, Kick, Punch Workout Guides			
Exercises	**Beginner**	**Intermediate**	**Advanced**
Jumping Jacks	10 - 30	30 - 50	50 - 100
Wind Mills, 4 count	5 - 15	15 - 30	30 - 80
Snap Kick, each leg	10 - 30	30 - 60	60 - 100
Side Punch Drill, 4 count	10 - 30	30 - 60	60 - 100
Toe Raisers, 4 count	20 - 40	40 - 70	70 - 100
Run 1 Mile	11:00 - 18:00	8:00 - 11:00	5:00 - 8:00
Run 2 Miles	16:00 - 30:00	14:00 - 16:00	10:00 - 14:00

Learn to see in another's calamity the ills that you should avoid.

- Thomas Jefferson

Chapter Nineteen

Abdominal Strength Training

The real investment is planning and executing your own fitness program as if you were commanding a military operation and your life and the lives of others depended upon it because they do.
– Lt. Col. Bob Weinstein, USAR, (ret.)

We see those ads and commercials all the time offering you the opportunity to get your very own six-pack abs just by buying and using this gadget or that gadget or this or that supplement, and mostly within a very brief period of time ranging from 24 hours to 3 months. These gadgets are predominantly and purportedly focusing on the abdominal region and promise that you, too, will lose inches of fat off of your waist, combined with proper diet. Do they work? Will you end up with visible, defined, washboard abs by focusing on exercising your abdominal region? No! It's a myth that any exercise focused on a specific body part will result in the loss of body fat in that specific area. For more details on exercise and diet fairy tales, see the chapter on myths.

Please keep in mind that it is not necessarily a healthy state to have the level of body fat to see clearly defined abs. Just remember that your body also needs body fat. Not enough body fat and too much body fat are both unhealthy states. See the chapter on "Fitness Goals and Progress Measurement" for calculation of your BMI or Body Mass Index.

With these abdominal region exercises below, you will achieve excellent abdominal strength and will also strengthen the surrounding muscles as well, such as lower abs, obliques, hips, thighs and hip flexors. Your cost? Well, the cost of this book. Of course, the real investment is planning and executing your own fitness program as if you were commanding a military operation and your life and the lives of others depended upon it. Guess what? Your life and the lives of others, who see you and get inspired to do the same, do depend upon the implementation of a consistent exercise and proper eating program.

CRUNCHES

Let's get started on the road to that six-pack that you so desire and begin with crunches.

Keep in mind that there are really 1,001 ways to perform this and other body weight exercises. Here's how we will perform the crunch. Get on your back. Take your hands and clasp them behind your head, bend your knees and bring your heels close to your butt. Lift those shoulders up off the ground or floor and lower them again. Start off with 10 to 20 reps per set and work your way up to 50 to 100 or more per set. This is just a slight motion. Concentrate on contracting those abs. Do enough of these and you will notice that the crunch can really work those abs. The motion should be smooth without going too fast.

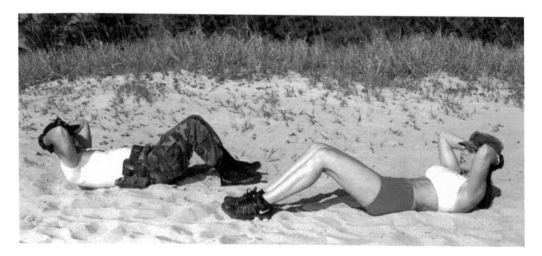

RAPID FIRE CRUNCHES

I know! I know! I just said perform your crunches smooth without going too fast. Well, I changed my mind. Let's add a rapid fire crunch to your arsenal. Now I'm not sure I really need to explain "rapid fire," but I'm going to do it anyway. A rapid fire crunch is the equivalent of a sprint; but you are performing crunches. The command to start after getting into the crunch position is, "On your mark! Get set! Go!" Now rapidly perform those crunches and count out loud! Perform anywhere from 20 to 50 per set. After a couple of sets of rapid fire abs, you will feel those abs working. Hey, you know what? You just added a cardio workout while performing crunches. I'll bet that makes you so excited that you'll get right down and do another set to celebrate!

CRUNCHES WITH LEG RAISED AND EXTENDED

Now we're going to vary the crunch by doing crunches with one leg extended off of the ground. Start out with the right leg extended six inches off of the ground and hands still clasped behind your head. We'll practice a set of 30 reps on each leg. Here's how. Perform 10 crunches with the leg six inches off of the ground, then 10 with the leg half way up, then 10 with the leg reaching for the sky. Now switch off and do the same with the left leg or simply switch legs between each set of 10 reps with each leg.

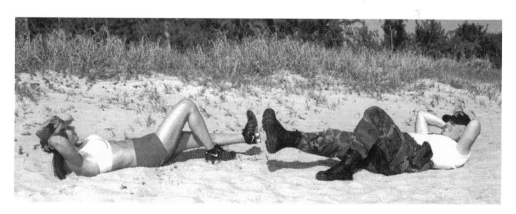

FOUR-COUNT-LEG-LEVERS

Let's move on to the four-count-leg-levers. You're still on your back. This time place your hands with palms facing down on the ground and arms extended at the sides of your body to stabilize the lower back and your head raised. The starting position is with legs raised six inches off of the ground and together. Now here's the four-count. ONE – raise the legs up to about 36 inches off of the ground. TWO – spread the legs while still raised at the 36 inch level. THREE – bring the legs back together while still at the 36 inch level. FOUR – back down to the position 6 inches off of the ground. This exercise also works the hip flexors, lower abs and lower back. Do 10 reps per set with multiple sets. Start off with no more than five reps per set if you notice a lot of strain on the lower back and work up to 10 reps.

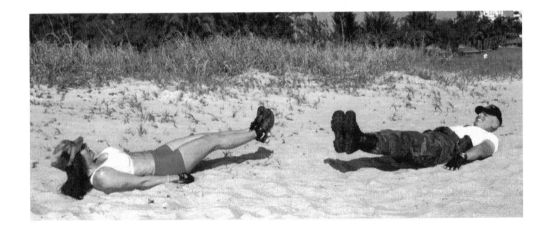

FLUTTER KICKS

You're still on your back with arms extended on the sides of your body and palms facing down to stabilize the lower back and your head raised. Raise up both of your legs in a staggered position (one leg is higher than the other) with a slight bend in the knees. This is a four count exercise. With each count you will simply switch the leg positions which makes it look like a scissor move, not a bicycle pedaling. This is your leg movement for the count: ONE, scissor move; TWO, scissor move; THREE, scissor move; FOUR, scissor move. Here's how you count the reps: One, two, three, ONE; one, two, three, TWO; one, two, three, THREE, one, two, three, FOUR; one, two, three, FIVE. Do five to ten reps per set with multiple sets and very brief rests between sets.

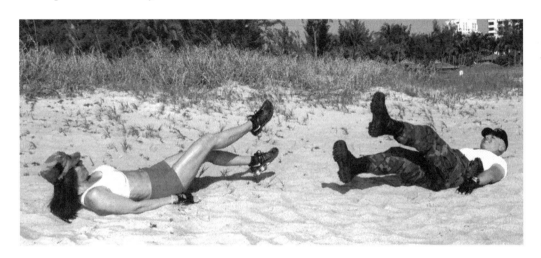

SIT-UPS

Don't you think about getting up! We're not done, yet. Let's get them all done. The next one is a little more advanced. The next exercise is the sit-up. This exercise is one of the events in the Army Physical Fitness Test. If you're not used to doing a sit-up, those muscles will need some developing. Your motion should be smooth, no jerking your body up. If you can't go all the way up, start out by going as far as you can. You're on your back with hands clasped behind your head and feet a little less than shoulder width apart with bent knees and feet on the ground. Curl your body up to the point where you have brought your body out of the range of exertion. When you're out of the range of exertion and it becomes easy, then lower it back down in the starting position with the same smooth motion. That's one repetition. Perform 10 to 50 reps per set. If you are having difficulties, use a slow count until you develop those muscles.

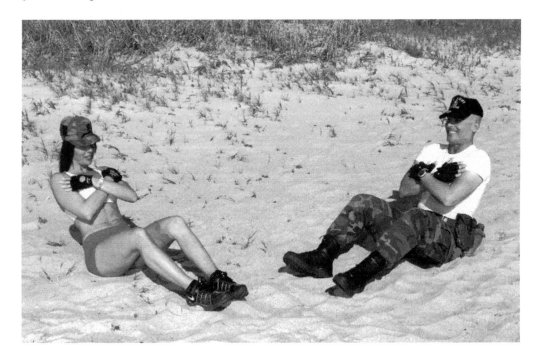

REACH FOR THE TOES

You're on your back. Raise both your legs together as high as you can. Now with your arms extended, palms facing down and hands close together, reach for your toes and then back to the starting position with shoulders and back on the ground. If you can touch your toes, that's great! If not, just do the best you can and keep working and don't give up. The muscles are still enjoying the benefit of being worked. Make sure you are raising the shoulders ever so slightly when reaching for your toes.

ALTERNATING ELBOW CRUNCH

Here's another great abdominal exercise. We'll call it the alternating elbow crunch. You're on your back. Your hands are clasped behind your head. Your left leg is bent. Cross your right leg over your left knee. Take your left elbow and reach for your right knee and back down. That is one rep. Use a smooth motion. Don't be concerned if you can't reach your leg with your elbow. Do the best you can. Remember, by performing the exercise you are working those muscles! Now switch off by crossing your left leg over your right knee, reach for your knee with your right elbow and do it again.

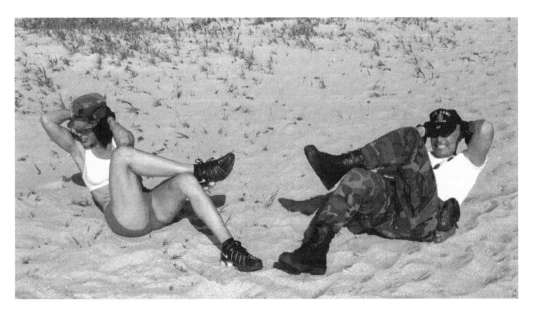

ATOMIC SIT-UPS

It's time for atomic sit-ups. Yeah. That's right! We're going nuclear! Laydown on your back with legs extended and arms extended to your sides. The starting position is with legs six inches off the ground. Now pull your knees and your chest to the middle where you are in a position balanced on your butt. Your body is briefly in that jack-knifed position. As you move into this position, bend your elbows so that your hands are at your shoulders. Now lower your legs back out to the extended position six inches off of the ground with your arms extended. That's one rep. Perform 10 to 40 reps per set.

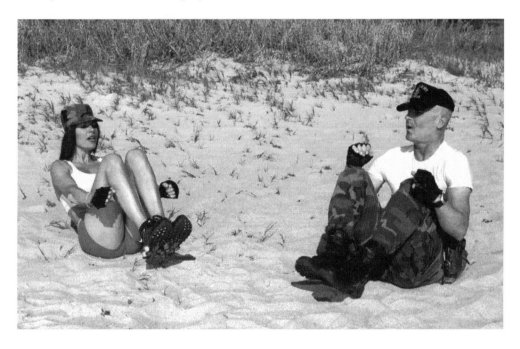

Six-pack Abs Workout Guide Reps			
	Beginner	**Intermediate**	**Advanced**
Crunches	10 - 50	50 - 120	120 - 300
Rapid Fire Crunches	10 - 30	30 - 60	60 - 150
Crunches with Leg Raised	10 - 60	60 - 120	120 - 320
4-count Leg Levers	0 - 10	10 - 20	20 - 40
Flutter Kicks	3 - 10	10 - 30	30 - 60
Sit-ups, reps	0 - 10	10 - 40	40 - 100
Reach for the toes!	10 - 40	40 - 60	60 - 100
Alternating Elbow Crunch-up	5 - 10	10 - 30	30 - 60
Atomic Sit-ups	5 - 10	10 - 30	30 - 60

CONCLUSION

Take Action Now

"The chief cause of failure and unhappiness is trading what you want most for what you want now." - Zig Ziglar

You have now been equipped to take charge of your eating and exercise routines and to design your values-based lifestyle so that you really can be all that you want to be and get all that you can out of life, to your benefit and to the benefit of others around you. By practicing these basics, you will bring about more positive change in the coming months and years than most people do in a lifetime.

Never give up. Develop that healthy habit of implementing change and taking action on all your worthy goals, regardless of set-backs or obstacles or struggles with oneself. No matter how many times you may fall or are delayed in accomplishing change in your life that you truly desire, get back up and keep moving with confidence. Here are some of the back-to-basics keys to achieving a healthy and joyful life.

1. Improve your character every day and choose what's right over what's comfortable.
2. Take inventory of your lifestyle regularly.
3. Spend some quiet time every day.
4. Read just a little every day about improving your character, relationships and lifestyle.
5. Manage your weight.
6. Beware of any quick-fix offers.
7. Use difficulties as a catalyst for change.
8. Be a positive influence on others.

9. Invite others to join you in your workouts.
10. Be a positive role model and voice of change in your community, city and state.
11. Measure your progress.
12. Have a close personal relationship with the creator.
13. Be successful.
14. Eat for performance and energy.
15. Exercise the complete body and the heart.
16. Volunteer to help others even if it's just one hour per week.
17. Be a role model for our youth.
18. Always be kind and compassionate.

Challenge to Change Lifestyle Contract

1. I want to change the following lifestyle habit:
2. I want to change this habit for the following reasons:
3. If I changed this habit, I feel I would:
4. The results of the change by me:
5. I plan to make this change in the following manner (list specific steps or action plans for creating this change).
6. My plan for evaluating my success will include:

I agree to discuss further my change in my lifestyle habit with

_____ by _____ (date).

I agree to discuss with _____ his/her success

in changing a lifestyle habit by _____ (date).

_____
Signature of partner

Complete Overview of Exercises

Exercises	Beginner	Intermediate	Advanced
Upper Body			
Regular Push-up, reps	2 - 20	20 - 30	30 - 100
Wide Push-up, reps	2 - 15	15 - 25	25 - 60
Tricep Push-up, reps	2 - 8	8 - 20	20 - 50
4-count Push-up, reps	2 - 5	8 - 20	20 - 40
Knee Push-ups, 45 Degrees, reps	10 - 20	20 - 60	60 - 100
Knee Push-ups, 90 Degrees, reps	10 - 20	20 - 60	60 - 100
Regular Pull-up, reps	0 - 5	5 - 10	10 - 25
Reverse Pull-up, reps	0 - 5	5 - 15	15 - 30
Hands-together Tricep Pull-up, reps	0 - 3	3 - 10	10 - 20
Extra Wide Pull-up, reps	0 - 2	2 - 5	5 - 15
Cliffhangers, reps	0 - 2	2 - 10	10 - 20
Assisted Pull-ups, reps	3 - 10	10 - 30	30 - 40
Straight Leg Inclines, reps	2 - 8	8 - 20	20 - 40
Regular Dips, reps	5 - 15	15 -40	40 - 100
Leg Extended Dips, reps (each leg)	5 - 10	10 - 20	20 - 40
Upper Body with Resistance Band			
Bicep Curls, reps	5 - 30	30 - 60	60 - 100
Upright Row, reps	5 - 40	40 - 60	60 - 100
Shoulder Press, reps	3 - 10	10 - 15	15 - 40
Front Raise, reps	5 - 10	10 - 15	15 - 20
Side Lateral Raise, reps	5 - 10	10 - 15	15 - 20
Standing Row, reps	10 - 40	40 - 70	70 - 100
Standing Triceps Push, reps	5 - 10	10 - 20	20 - 30
Reverse Curls, reps	4 - 15	15 - 20	20 - 40
Partner Assisted Standing Arm Curl, reps	10 - 20	20 - 30	30 - 60

	Beginner	Intermediate	Advanced
Lower Body Exercises			
Squats, reps	20 - 40	40 - 100	100 - 200
Standing Lunges, reps, each leg	5 - 20	20 - 60	60 - 100
Dirty Dogs, reps, each leg	5 - 10	10 - 40	40 - 80
Leg Thrusts, reps, each leg	5 - 20	20 - 50	50 - 80
Standing Crunches, reps, each leg	10 - 30	30 - 60	60 - 100
Alternating Side Leg Raise (Lift)	10 - 15	15 - 30	30 - 70
Other Exercises			
Jumping Jacks	10 - 30	30 - 50	50 - 100
Wind Mills, 4 count	5 - 15	15 - 30	30 - 80
Snap Kick, each leg	10 - 30	30 - 60	60 - 100
Side Punch Drill, 4 count	10 - 30	30 - 60	60 - 100
Toe Raisers, 4 count	20 - 40	40 - 70	70 - 100
Run			
Run 1 Mile	11:00 - 18:00	8:00 - 11:00	5:00 - 8:00
Run 2 Miles	16:00 - 30:00	14:00 - 16:00	10:00 - 14:00
Abs and Others			
Crunches	10 - 50	50 - 120	120 - 300
Rapid Fire Crunches	10 - 30	30 - 60	60 - 150
Crunches with Leg Raised	10 - 60	60 - 120	120 - 320
4-count Leg Levers	0 - 10	10 - 20	20 - 40
Flutter Kicks	3 - 10	10 - 30	30 - 60
Sit-ups, reps	0 - 10	10 - 40	40 - 100
Reach for the toes!	10 - 40	40 - 60	60 - 100
Alternating Elbow Crunch-up	5 - 10	10 - 30	30 - 60
Atomic Sit-ups	5 - 10	10 - 30	30 - 60

Contact Info:
Lt. Col. Bob Weinstein, USAR-Ret.
Beach Boot Camp Instructor and Motivational Speaker
www.TheHealthColonel.com
954-636-5351
TheHealthColonel@BeachBootCamp.net

Mailing address:
757 SE 17th Street, #267
Fort Lauderdale, FL
33316

LEARNING
RESOURCES

Official Website of Lt. Col. Bob Weinstein, USAR, (ret.)
TheHealthColonel.com

The Health Colonel™ Workout DVD
Beach Boot Camp Upper Body Blast
ShopColonelBob.com

Six Keys to Permanent Weight Loss and Eight Ways to Get and Stay in Shape
ShopColonelBob.com

American Dietetic Association
Eatright.org

Micronutrients Research for Optimum Health
Lpi.oregonstate.edu

American Diabetes Association
Diabetes.org

American Heart Association
Americanheart.org

Covenant House,
Great place to volunteer and help our homeless and runaway youth.
Covenanthouse.org

U.S. Naval Sea Cadets
Excellent leadership and life skills training for 12 to 17-year-olds.
Seacadets.org

National Coalition for the Homeless
Show compassion. Help the homeless.
Nationalhomeless.org

Veterans Administration
Help the veterans.
Va.gov

U. S. Army
GoArmy.com

Index

H

I

Z

Products By Lt. Col. Bob Weinstein, USAR-Ret.

Get Your Priorities Straight - Audio CD and MP3 Download
Put an end to indecisiveness and take back control of your life. Learn to move out with confidence and purpose. Learn to overcome life obstacles. Discover your true life priorities and how to implement them. Find out how to reinvent your life into the true you that is already inside and waiting to be allowed to live life to the fullest. Discover the ultimate law of happiness and learn how to apply it today.

Quotes to Live By - Paperback and EBook
My personal journey to seek out wisdom and improvement in my life and the lives of others has resulted in this collection of quotes. May they inspire you or someone you know to be a better person and always take the high road when faced with challenging decisions. The journey is still in progress for me and will last a lifetime.

Six Keys to Permanent Weight-loss - Audio CD and MP3 Download
Join the Fitness and Beach Boot Camp Instructor, Lt. Col. Bob Weinstein, USAR, (ret.), on his over 60 minute journey to successful and permanent weight loss, delivered with enthusiasm, humor and high energy. You will tap into the vast experience of the Health Colonel. You will talk, think and eat yourself lean after following Colonel Weinstein's straightforward, no-nonsense, Six Keys to Permanent Weight Loss.

Boot Camp Fitness For All Shapes and Sizes: Complete Manual
Put on your commander's hat. You are about to take charge of your health. This book is a health and fitness blueprint to get America back in shape, keep Americans from dying of ill health and keep Americans strong. A combination of self-help, right eating, exercising, how to start a fitness boot camp, weight loss as well as guidance on how to lead a values-based life to the benefit of others and our society. Lots of exercise photos. Paperback and EBook

Eight Secrets to Longevity, Health and Fitness - Audio CD and MP3
An exciting journey to empower and educate you to take charge of your health and eating habits. Put on your commander's hat and take charge of your all those body parts that may not be firm as they used to. Delivered with enthusiasm, humor and high energy. You will tap into the vast experience of the Health Colonel. A Straight-forward, no-nonsense, back-to-basics approach to exercise and eating.

Products By Lt. Col. Bob Weinstein, USAR-Ret.

Beach Boot Camp Upper Body Blast - DVD Video

Suitable for all fitness levels and excellent for group exercise instruction. This video is much more than those follow-along workout routines on the market. It includes great workout tips, humor, great beach scenes and inspirational and motivational guidance all wrapped into this dynamic 29 minute program. The workout is filmed on Fort Lauderdale Beach in Florida. Join him with his group class as he equips and empowers you to take your workout to the next level. Both natural body weight exercises as well as some using an inexpensive rubber resistance band are demonstrated.

Weight Loss - Twenty Pounds in Ten Weeks - Paperback and EBook

Weight Loss and weight management book with a ten week exercise and eating plan to lose twenty pounds. Full of easy-to-use tools to organize and implement the program: exercise photos, ten week exercise chart, 1,200 and 1,600 calorie menus, calorie burn charts, workout log, food diary and more. The author, Lt. Col. Weinstein has been featured on the History Channel. TheHealthColonel.com

For more info call toll free 888-768-9892.

Don't curse the darkness, light a candle.

- Chinese proverb

Speaker Topics as Keynotes and Workshops by Lt. Col. Weinstein

The Eight Universal Laws of Getting and Staying in Shape

Over 3,000 Americans die of heart disease, cancer and stroke. Over eighty percent of these deaths are lifestyle related. Your organization will make sure that their employees do not become a lifestyle-related casualty of this war on fighting disease and maintaining good health.

Six Keys to Permanent Weight Loss

50 % of Americans are overweight, 33% are obese, and as many as 40% of women and 25% of men are trying to lose weight at any given time. We have a serious crisis of overeating and leading a sedentary lifestyle. This topic is designed to equip the audience with the necessary strategic and tactical knowledge to conquer these health issues.

Cost Effective Wellness Programs for Small, Medium and Large Businesses

According to the Centers for Disease Control, more than 75% of employer health care costs and productivity losses are related to employee lifestyle choices. Other studies have revealed that about 20% are responsible for 80%of the costs. You will be given the necessary tools to immediately implementa cost effective wellness program that significantly improves the health and performance of your employees.

How to Combat Childhood Obesity

The percentage of our youth who are overweight has tripled since the early 1970's. Col. Weinstein addresses the six "secrets" to combating the youth health crisis. We are killing our children and preparing them to have serious health issues early in life. You will be pointed in the right direction to guide and inspire our youth to lead healthy and happy lives.

Give-up vs. Take-charge Talk

Getting back on track with performance based living is a matter of how we think. You will learn how to identify and eliminate what Col. Weinstein calls give-up talk and replace it with take-charge talk when it comes to healthy living.

Get Back Up and Catch Your Second Wind!

We've all heard the expression "Catch your second wind!" Unfortunately, the vast majority of people don't even know what the second wind feels like and there is a reason for this. Ninety percent usually give-up as soon as the first difficulties or challenges occur. Col. Weinstein will give you those insights necessary to take you and your worthy goals into the realm of the second wind and keep up that momentum.

Values and Character Matter Most

There is no exception. Values and character do matter most and are foundational for sound relationships in the business world and in our family lives.

Whether you are interested in furthering your career, building high-performance teams or showing our youth or adults the way to lead a truly values-based life, this is the topic for you and your organization.

About the Author

Born in Washington, D.C., Lt. Col. Bob Weinstein grew up in Virginia and spent 20 years in Berlin, Germany; he is retired from the Army Reserve as a Lieutenant Colonel with 30 years of service and spent about half of that time as a military instructor with the Command & General Staff College.

He has been featured on radio and television, among others, on the History Channel and Fox Sports Net as well as in various publications such as the Washington Times, RAZOR magazine and the Herald.

His background is unique and diverse, including: military instructor, attorney, motivational speaker, wellness coach, certified corporate trainer, and certified personal trainer. He is also fluent in German and English.

He is a popular motivational speaker at corporate events and banquets and conducts military-style workouts on Fort Lauderdale Beach utilizing strength, cardio, flexibility and agility training -- both in personal training and group sessions.

He strongly believes in the importance of giving back to the community. Col. Weinstein volunteers his time for homeless and run-away kids at the Covenant House and also devotes time to training youth who are members of the US Naval Sea Cadet Corps.

He is a member of the National Speakers Association and the American Council on Exercise, and is currently working on a book about personal development, health and fitness. Some of his previous clients as a guest speaker include: Sony, DHL, American Express, KPMG, AOL Latin America, IBM, AARP, SmithBarney, Green Bay Packers and Humana.

To purchase additional copies of this book or other products by Lt. Col. Bob Weinstein, USAR-Ret call our toll free order number at:
1-888-768-9892

or visit his website at:
www.TheHealthColonel.com

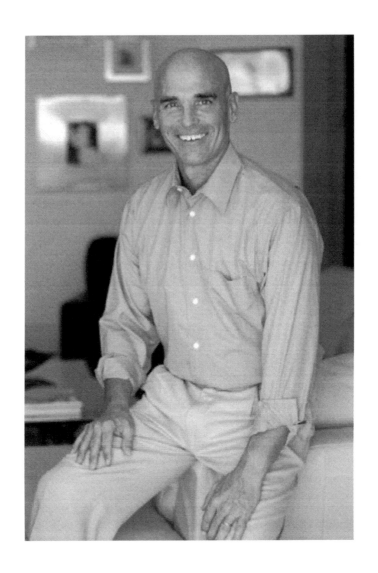

Lt. Col. Bob Weinstein, USAR-Ret.
Fort Lauderdale, Florida

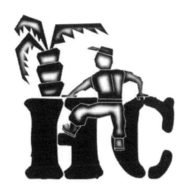

THEHEALTHCOLONEL.COM

**CHANGING THE WAY PEOPLE
THINK ABOUT HEALTH.**

QUICK ORDER FORM

Fax orders: 866-481-2804. Send this form.

Telephone orders: Call 888-768-9892 toll-free

Email orders: thehealthcolonel@beachbootcamp.net

Postal orders: The Health Colonel, Lt. Col. Bob Weinstein, USAR-Ret., 757 SE 17th Street, #267, Fort Lauderdale, FL 33316, Telephone 954-636-5351

Please send the following books, audio CDs, DVDs:

Please send more FREE information on:

❑   Other books   ❑   Speaking/seminars

❑   Fitness Boot Camp   ❑   Mailing Lists

Name:

Address:

City: State: Zip:

Telephone:

Email address:

Sales tax: Please add Florida sales tax for products shipped to Florida addresses.

Shipping:
U.S.: $4.50 for first book, CD or DVD and $2.50 for each additional product.
International: $9.50 for first product; $5.50 for each additional product (estimate).

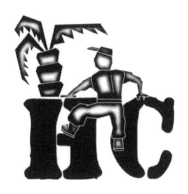

THEHEALTHCOLONEL.COM

CHANGING THE WAY PEOPLE THINK ABOUT HEALTH.

QUICK ORDER FORM

Fax orders: 866-481-2804. Send this form.

Telephone orders: Call 888-768-9892 toll-free

Email orders: thehealthcolonel@beachbootcamp.net

Postal orders: The Health Colonel, Lt. Col. Bob Weinstein, USAR-Ret., 757 SE 17th Street, #267, Fort Lauderdale, FL 33316, Telephone 954-636-5351

Please send the following books, audio CDs, DVDs:

Please send more FREE information on:

❑　　　　Other books　　　❑　　　　Speaking/seminars

❑　　　　Fitness Boot Camp　❑　　　　Mailing Lists

Name:

Address:

City:　　　　　　　　　　　　State:　　　Zip:

Telephone:

Email address:

Sales tax: Please add Florida sales tax for products shipped to Florida addresses.

•

Shipping:
U.S.: $4.50 for first book, CD or DVD and $2.50 for each additional product.
International: $9.50 for first product; $5.50 for each additional product (estimate).

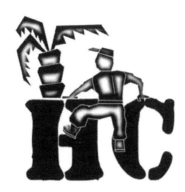

THEHEALTHCOLONEL.COM

**CHANGING THE WAY PEOPLE
THINK ABOUT HEALTH.**

QUICK ORDER FORM

Fax orders: 866-481-2804. Send this form.

Telephone orders: Call 888-768-9892 toll-free

Email orders: thehealthcolonel@beachbootcamp.net

Postal orders: The Health Colonel, Lt. Col. Bob Weinstein, USAR-Ret., 757 SE 17th Street, #267, Fort Lauderdale, FL 33316, Telephone 954-636-5351

Please send the following books, audio CDs, DVDs:

Please send more FREE information on:

❑　　　Other books　　　❑　　　Speaking/seminars

❑　　　Fitness Boot Camp　　　❑　　　Mailing Lists

Name:

Address:

City:　　　　　　　　　　　　State:　　　Zip:

Telephone:

Email address:

Sales tax: Please add Florida sales tax for products shipped to Florida addresses.

Shipping:
U.S.: $4.50 for first book, CD or DVD and $2.50 for each additional product.
International: $9.50 for first product; $5.50 for each additional product (estimate).

Made in the USA
Lexington, KY
10 June 2010